This Book Is For You If...

☑ You already suffer from gout (and want to relieve the symptoms)

☑ You think you may be suffering from gout (and want to find out more)

☑ Someone you love, either a family member of a friend, has gout

☑ You want the best possible advice on the causes of gout, and what to eat and drink to get rid of it as quickly as possible.

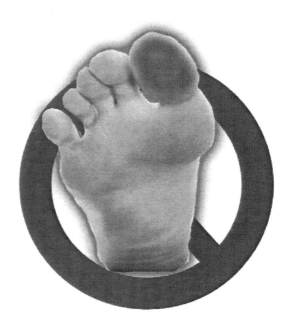

Here's What Readers Say About Dr Spira's Books...

'...offers instead a sensible, scientifically based programme...'
"A really common sense approach to successful slimming. Without the unnatural use of pills and diet sheets, it offers instead a sensible, scientifically based programme of eating that could help even the weakest willed to take off weight. Most important it helps encourage an eating pattern that will keep your weight loss permanent."
The Lady

'...excellent book...'
"An excellent book. This should be read not only by interested laymen but also by any professional person involved in dealing with overweight individuals."
Modern Medicine

'...worth trying...'
"The method does not take iron willpower, and it does become a permanent eating habit. It is a method which most overweight people would find worth trying."
The Daily Telegraph

'...recommended to every person...'
"This is one of the finest slim books on the subject which has caused tremendous anxiety to millions of people the world over who are suffering from the evil effects of obesity and are unable to follow a strict regimen of diet. The author shows here how to establish successful eating patterns with only a little self-control and how to remain slim as well as healthy. The volume is recommended to every person who is either having a slimming problem or is a potential candidate for the same."
Nutrition

'...a sensible programme...'
"Offers a sensible programme of eating that will help even the weakest willed to take off weight."
Finchley Press

'...Dr Spira really knows his stuff.'
"One of the best books on slimming and nutrition. Dr Spira really knows his stuff."
London Evening News

'...full of sensible information...'
"An excellent book, full of sensible information and advice for any serious would-be slimmer of any age who wants to understand what losing weight is really all about."
Update

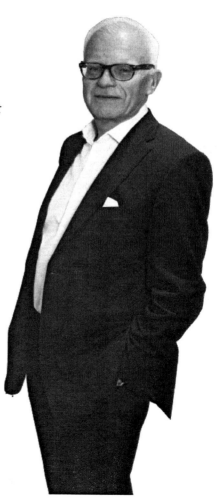

'Good advice...'
"Good advice for dieters"
Women's Weekly

'...contain(s) the secret of successful slimming.'
"This book genuinely does contain the secret of successful slimming"
Bracknell News

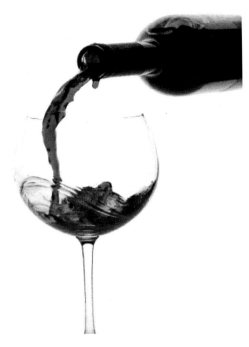

"Be temperate in wine,
in eating,
girls, and cloth,
or the Gout
will seize you
and plague you."

Benjamin Franklin 1706 - 1790

A Quick Note From Nick Wrathall,
Editor, *Goutbusters*

You never forget the first time you have a serious attack of gout...

I was in my late thirties when I woke up one morning and was horrified to discover my right leg below the knee red, swollen and agonising.

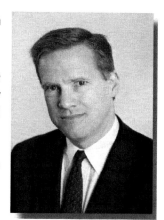

What was happening? Was it life-threatening? Why is it so painful?

All these questions were racing through my mind as I staggered to my doctor.

The worst part? The pain was so intense, and I limped so slowly, that I was overtaken on the pavement by an elderly lady with a walker!

Once I arrived at the doctor's surgery, his diagnosis was immediate: a simple blood test soon confirmed the doctor's suspicions that I was suffering from gout, and I received a prescription of 'weapons-grade' NSAIDs, which fortunately worked quickly.

But I still had a lot of questions...

What is gout? What triggered attacks? And most important of all, how could I prevent gout attacks and relieve the symptoms of gout pain should it strike again?

In other words, the best diet, medication and lifestyle choices to make sure I didn't have to endure the agony of gout, or the greater pain of unknown side-effects from medication.

Fortunately, Dr Spira, the leading UK expert on gout, had all the answers.

Just as well because there are now two million UK citizens who are suffering.

Inside *Goutbusters*, Dr Spira explains exactly what gout is, how to recognise the symptoms of gout, and the treatment options available to you, including the simple, proven and practical ways to prevent gout attacks from occurring.

You'll also discover why it's vitally important to treat your gout correctly, and treat it early, plus the life-threatening conditions you could suffer if your gout isn't treated.

Goutbusters also provides you with sections on alternative and complementary medicine (and how they can help you), the latest cutting-edge research into gout treatment, case studies of how people have tackled and overcome gout (including my own 'gout-busting' treatment plan), and much more besides.

You'll even get a *'food traffic light plan'*, which shows you which foods trigger gout attacks (to avoid eating), the ones to be careful about, and the foods you can eat without fear.

Goutbusters is divided into five sections: the first three parts give you all the facts you need on gout in layman's terms, the fourth section gives you additional resources you can use (if you want to find out more about gout), and the fifth section gives you the scientific and medical reports and proof to back up everything Dr Spira says.

Finally, thank you for getting this book, and I hope you find it interesting, informative and an effective tool for fighting your gout – and regaining control of your health and life...

Time to start your gout pain-relief journey.

About Dr Michael Spira

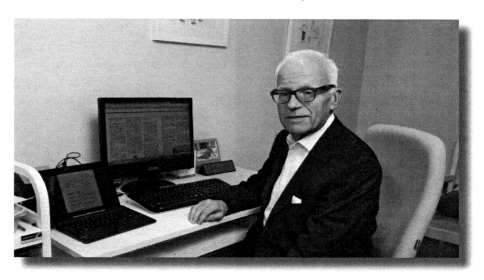

Dr Michael Spira, MB BS MRCS LRCP, qualified as a doctor at London's St Bartholomew's Hospital. After initially specialising in eye surgery, he is now a GP and Medical Director in a private clinic in central London.

Dr Spira is one of the UK's top diet and obesity experts and the author of several diet books including *How to Lose Weight Without Really Dieting* (Penguin) amongst others.

He was for many years a medical consultant at a leading group of wellness clinics where advice on diet and lifestyle were key issues, and is also a member of the National Obesity Forum.

Besides his many books and articles, Dr Spira is regularly featured as a guest on national TV and radio including as medical expert on **BBC1's Kilroy**, **ITV's GMTV** and **ITV's The Gloria Hunniford Show**.

He is currently Medical Director of The Smart Clinics which provide integrated healthcare in South Kensington, Notting Hill and Wandsworth.

Dr Spira's publications include...

- *Basic Health Education* (with Vincent Irwin) (Longman 1977)
- *How To Lose Weight Without Really Dieting* (Penguin 1978, revised edition 1988)
- *The No Diet Book* (Fontana 1982)
- *The 3D Diet* (Corgi 1984)
- *Understanding Menopause* (Hawker Publications 1987)
- *Understanding Nutrition* (Hawker Publications 1996)
- *Angina* (Hawker Publications 1996)
- *How To Lose Weight Now And Forever* (2004)
- *The Chelsea Diet* (2006)

Dr Spira is also a contributor to...

- Everyman's Encyclopaedia (Dent)
- BMA Complete Family Health Encyclopaedia (Dorling-Kindersley 1990)
- The Mind (Readers Digest 2003)

> "The best medicine I know for rheumatism is to thank the Lord that it ain't gout."
>
> Josh Billings

Acknowledgements

Any worthwhile endeavour is never completed alone, and this book is no exception, with several people worthy of mention in its drafting and compilation, not least my family and friends.

I'd like to thank Dr Michael Spira for all his hard work in writing the bulk of this book…

I'd also like to thank Chris and Zara at Filament Publishing for their typesetting and editing expertise…

But most of all, I'd like to thank you, Dear Reader, for investing your time and money in this book. I sincerely hope your gout pain is relieved thanks to what you find in these pages.

And finally, a special word of thanks to – sadly – two absent friends who believed in me when no one else did…

To Jerry R. Wilson, word of mouth marketer, customerologist and confidence-booster extraordinaire.

And the last word, as ever, to 'JG', one of a kind, sophisticated motivator, teacher, father confessor and 'always the first to copy the best'.

My thoughts and gratitude are with you.

Do you suffer from gout? Then you're in exalted company. As you'll see in *Goutbusters*, gout is no respecter of class or background, with over two million UK sufferers. Members of the famous gout sufferers' club include:

- Alexander the Great
- Charlemagne
- Henry VIII
- Queen Anne
- Dr Samuel Johnson
- Christopher Columbus
- Nostradamus
- Leonardo da Vinci
- Michaelangelo
- John Milton
- Sir Isaac Newton
- Alfred, Lord Tennyson
- Thomas Jefferson
- Benjamin Franklin
- Ludwig van Beethoven
- Daniel Defoe
- Sitting Bull
- Benjamin Disraeli
- King George IV
- Karl Marx
- William Waldorf Astor
- Neville Chamberlain
- Dylan Thomas
- Sir Laurence Olivier
- Sir Alec Guinness
- Jared Leto
- David Wells (ex-MLB Baseball player)
- Maurice Cheeks (ex-NBA Basketball player)
- Harry Kewell (Ex-Australian and Leeds United footballer)
- Luciano Pavarotti
- James Belushi
- Dick Cheney

And...you... *To see how to 'leave the club', please turn over the page...*

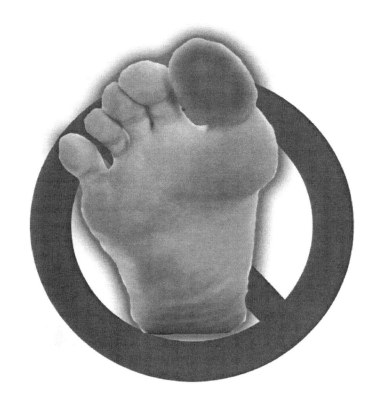

G⊘UTBUSTERS

Dr Michael Spira
in conversation with
Nick Wrathall

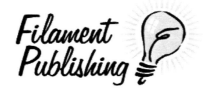

Published by
Filament Publishing Ltd
16, Croydon Road, Waddon, Croydon,
Surrey, CR0 4PA, United Kingdom
Telephone +44 (0)20 8688 2598
Fax +44 (0)20 7183 7186
info@filamentpublishing.com
www.filamentpublishing.com

ISBN 978-1-910125-65-6

Printed by Berforts Information Press
Stevenage & Hastings

If medical advice or other expert assistance is required, the services
of a competent professional person should be sought.

Contents

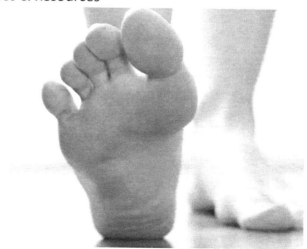

GOUT, n.
A physician's name for the rheumatism
of a rich patient.   Ambrose Bierce

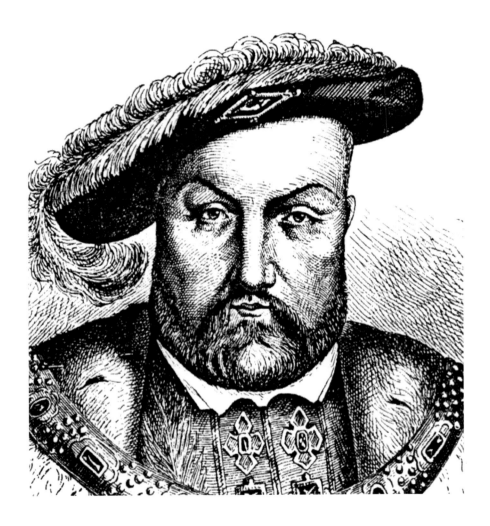

Introduction: Broad overview

Gout is one of the oldest known diseases in human history. In fact, it used to be called 'the disease of kings' because it was associated with rich living. Notable sufferers in history include King Henry VIII, Benjamin Franklin and Goethe, so you're in exalted company!

Doctors believe that we're now in the midst of the third great gout epidemic of the Western world.

The reasons for the increase in the prevalence of gout in the past 50 years include:

- An increase in the prevalence of metabolic syndrome.

- A combination of the medical disorders that, when occuring together, increase the risk of developing cardiovascular disease and diabetes.

- This in turn reflects the increase in the average weight of the Western population.

During the first two great gout epidemics – those of the Roman and British empires - gout was associated mainly with drinking alcohol, and to a lesser extent with lead poisoning.

In the present epidemic, gout is largely associated with obesity.

Other factors include:

- An increase in the use of low-dose aspirin (but not high-dose aspirin)

- Diuretics (drugs that increase the amount of urine you pass)

- Other medications

- An increase in the number of organ transplants.

Gout is a type of arthritis that affects around 1-2% of the population, and

- It's the most common form of inflammatory arthritis in the elderly.

- It's often linked to being overweight, having a rich diet or drinking a lot of alcohol.

- The main form of treatment is usually with anti-inflammatory drugs.

The word gout comes from Latin *gutta* and also from old French gote meaning *"a drop"*.

Hundreds of years ago, it was thought that gout was caused by drops of viscous humors that seeped from blood into the joints. In fact, this is not as fanciful as it sounds.

An acute attack of gout is caused by uric acid that has been accumulating in your blood passing into a joint and forming deposits or crystals of uric acid.

Unlike all other forms of arthritis in which damage begins within joints, in gout damage begins outside the joint capsule.

Part 1

What exactly is gout?
(And how does it affect you?)

In this section, you'll discover...

- Why Gout is different from osteoarthritis and rheumatoid arthritis (page 20).

- The four different types of gout (which one do you have? Find out on page 23...).

- Are you more likely to get primary gout – or secondary gout? (See on page 25...)

- The foods you must not eat if you want to avoid agonising gout pain (page 26).

- How many of the 'unlucky 13' risk factors for gout apply to you. Discover for yourself on page 27...

- Can you drink alcohol and still avoid gout? (The answer may surprise you – page 28.)

- How likely are you to get gout? (The risk factors revealed on pages 31-32.)

- The diseases or conditions which can be mistaken for gout – do you have any of these, and not gout? Get the facts on pages 35, and much more...

Chapter 1

What is gout and what causes it?

In layman's terms, gout is a form of arthritis – a painful inflammation in one or more joints.

You've probably heard about the most common form of arthritis, known as osteoarthritis.

This is caused by the wear and tear that often affects many joints, especially weight bearing ones such as hips and knees, causing pain, loss of mobility of the joint(s) and often stiffness.

Sometimes joints become so badly worn that they need to be replaced, such as with hip replacement operations.

Another well-known but completely different type of arthritis is rheumatoid arthritis.

Rheumatoid arthritis is an auto-immune disease, in other words an abnormal immune response of the body against the joints. This is when the body thinks these joints are foreign bodies and therefore attacks them.

It's usually the small joints of the hands, feet and spine in the neck that are affected, but larger joints such as the shoulder and knee are sometimes affected. Rheumatoid arthritis sometimes affects not only joints but other body organs.

Gout is quite different to osteoarthritis and rheumatoid arthritis.

This is because it's often associated with high levels in the blood of a chemical called uric acid – a compound of carbon, nitrogen, oxygen, and hydrogen.

Gout arthritis is due to the formation within a joint or joints of crystals of a chemical called monosodium urate (MSU) monohydrate. These cause acute inflammation and, in time, tissue damage.

Gout is one of the most painful acute conditions that human beings can experience and is one of the first diseases ever to be recognised. Gout has, however, been known since ancient times.

- Historically, it has been referred to as *"the king of diseases and the disease of kings"* or *"rich man's disease"*.

- It was first described by Imhotep, an Egyptian who lived around 2650-2600 BC.

- It was also noted by the famous physician, Hippocrates, who lived around 460–377 BC. In fact it was Hippocrates who first made the distinction between gout and other forms of arthritis. He noted its absence in eunuchs and premenopausal women.

- In 1683 the eminent English physician, Thomas Sydenham, sometimes known as "the English Hippocrates", a gout sufferer for many years, was the first to give what is now a classic description of gout and its symptoms. He wrote:

"Gouty patients are, generally, either old men, or men who have so worn themselves out in youth as to have brought on a premature old age—of such dissolute habits none being more common than the premature and excessive indulgence in venery, and the like exhausting passions.

"The victim goes to bed and sleeps in good health. About 2 o'clock in the morning, he is awakened by a severe pain in the great toe; more rarely in the heel, ankle or instep.

"This pain is like that of a dislocation, and yet the parts feel as if cold water were poured over them. Then follows chills and shiver and a little fever.

"The pain which at first moderate becomes more intense. With its intensity the chills and shivers increase. After a time this comes to a full height, accommodating itself to the bones and ligaments of the tarsus and metatarsus.

"Now it is a violent stretching and tearing of the ligaments—now it is a gnawing pain and now a pressure and tightening. So exquisite and lively meanwhile is the feeling of the part affected, that it cannot bear the weight of bedclothes nor the jar of a person walking in the room."

- About 50 years ago, two doctors, Faires and MacCarty, bravely – some would say foolishly! - in an effort to study the role of MSU crystals in gout, injected their left knee joints with 20 mg of MSU crystals.

- Both men quickly developed an acute inflammation typical of a gout attack, and both experienced the most excruciating pain. When they had recovered, they wrote:

"At this point we were impressed by the accuracy of Sydenham's classic description of gout."

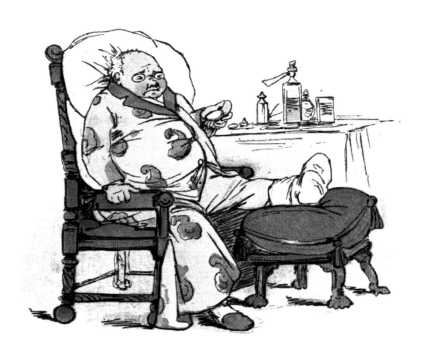

Chapter 2

Are there different types of gout?

There are four different types of gout. In fact, there are four different stages of the condition.

STAGE ONE: Asymptomatic hyperuricaemia

Hyperuricaemia is the name for higher than normal levels of uric acid in the blood.

Almost all patients with gout have hyperuricaemia, but...not all patients with hyperuricaemia have gout.

Most patients have high levels of uric acid in the blood for many years before having their first attack of gout. However current guidelines do not recommend treatment in the absence of actual gout, i.e. in the absence of symptoms of gout.

The condition of high uric acid levels *without* clinical gout is known as asymptomatic hyperuricaemia.

The risk of an attack of gout attack increases with increasing uric acid levels, but many patients have attacks with normal levels of uric acid and some patients never have an attack despite having very high levels of uric acid.

STAGE TWO: Acute gout

The second stage starts with a sudden attack of severe pain and swelling, most often in just one joint.

The attack typically lasts one to two weeks.

STAGE THREE: Intercritical gout

This stage is the time between attacks, and can last many months or even years.

During this time there is no joint pain or stiffness. However blood levels of uric acid are still high and patients may need treatment to prevent the next stage, chronic tophaceous gout.

STAGE FOUR: Chronic tophaceous gout

For some sufferers, gout can be an agonising recurring condition with multiple severe attacks that occur at short intervals, often with no completely pain-free period in between attacks.

This is called chronic gout and can lead to significant joint destruction and deformity – and sometimes may even be confused with other forms of chronic inflammatory arthritis, such as rheumatoid arthritis.

Often uric acid **tophi** are present.

In layman's terms, tophi are hard uric acid deposits under the skin, which can lead to the destruction of bone and cartilage destruction.

Tophi can be found around joints. They can also be found in the olecranon bursa – the small fluid-filled sac lined by synovial membrane with an inner layer of viscous fluid, that provides a cushion between bones and tendons and/or muscles around the elbow joint, and which helps to reduce friction between the bones and allows free movement.

Another site for tophi is the pinna (the visible part of the ear). With treatment, tophi can be dissolved and will usually completely disappear in time.

Another way of classifying gout is primary and secondary.

Primary gout

This occurs mainly in men aged 30-60 and presents itself with acute attacks.

Secondary gout

This is most often caused by diuretics (prescribed drugs that increase the production of urine), and occurs in older people of either sex. It is often associated with osteoarthritis.

"The gout is a complaint as arises from too much ease and comfort. If ever you're attacked with the gout, sir, jist you marry a widder as has got a good loud woice, with a decent notion of usin' it, and you'll never have the gout agin.... I can warrant it to drive away any illness as is caused by too much jollity."

Charles Dickens, The Pickwick Papers

Chapter 3

What are the risk factors for gout?
(And why does uric acid build up?)

You may have heard in the media about a substance called uric acid, and that it's a contributory factor to gout. But what exactly is it, and what does it do to cause gout?

- Uric acid is the relatively insoluble end-product of what's known as *'purine metabolism'*.

- Purines are organic compounds – some of which occur naturally in our bodies whilst others come from the food we eat.

- About two-thirds of uric acid comes from the breakdown of purines in our bodies, whilst around one-third comes from purines in our food.

Food sources of purine

The highest concentration of purines is in meat and meat products, especially liver and kidney.

Examples of foods high in purine content are: liver, beef kidneys, sweetbreads, anchovies, sardines, brains, meat extracts (e.g. Oxo, Bovril), mackerel, herring, scallops, game meats, beer (because of the yeast) and gravy.

So if you eat large amounts of certain types of meat and seafood, there's an increased risk of you suffering from gout.

Foods that contain a moderate amount of purines include beef, pork, poultry, many fish and seafood, cauliflower, spinach, asparagus, mushrooms, green peas, lentils, beans, dried peas, oatmeal, wheat bran and wheat germ.

On the bright side, plant-based foods are generally low in purines, and a higher level of consumption of dairy products is associated with a decreased risk. Purine-rich vegetables or protein are not associated with an increased risk of gout.

Uric Acid and Gout: The facts...

Around 70% of uric acid is excreted through your kidneys: the remainder passes out through the gut.

The commonest cause of hyperuricaemia (high blood levels of uric acid) is reduced renal (kidney) elimination from our bodies or increased production, or both.

As we've already seen, the metabolic syndrome and its components - obesity, high blood pressure, insulin resistance and high blood levels of fat - are very much associated with gout.

In fact, nearly two-thirds of patients with gout have the metabolic syndrome whereas only one-quarter of people without the metabolic syndrome have gout.

So, what are the important risk factors for gout?

Have a look at this list – how many of these factors apply to you?

−   A member of the male sex (almost 90% of gout sufferers are men)

−   Older age (over 35)

−   Genetic factors (mainly the reduced excretion of uric acid)

−   Metabolic syndrome (as described above)

−   Obesity (because of reduced excretion of uric acid)

−   High blood pressure (again, because of reduced excretion of uric acid)

- High levels of blood fat (because of reduced excretion of uric acid)

- Some diuretics (e.g. bendroflumethiazide, furosemide, bumetanide - because of reduced excretion of uric acid)

- Chronic kidney disease (because of reduced excretion of uric acid)

- Osteoarthritis (because of increased enhanced crystal formation)

- Dietary factors (because of increased production of uric acid)

- Excess purine-rich foods (including fructose and sugar-sweetened soft drinks)

- Excess alcohol consumption (especially beer)

Alcohol and the risk of gout

There's good news and bad news, so let's start with the bad...

The risk of developing gout is directly linked to alcohol consumption. But it depends on what kind of alcohol you drink.

As you might expect, the risk is highest for beer and spirits, but the good news is it's considerably less for wine.

In fact, a survey has shown that the daily consumption of a small glass of wine is not associated with an increased risk of developing gout.

However, sugar-sweetened soft drinks, especially those with fructose, increase the risk of gout.

On the other hand, dairy products, caffeinated and decaffeinated coffee seems to be protective (i.e. not a cause of gout).

But however *'clean-living'* you may be in terms of diet, liquid consumption and weight management, there's another key cause of gout to take into consideration: your genes.

Your genes and gout

Research has shown that gout often runs in families, but how much of this is due to lifestyle and how much due to genetic factors?

Current science hasn't yet found a definitive answer, although it's clear that some patients inherit a genetic predisposition to gout.

Prescribed drugs and gout

But that's not all... If you're taking prescription medication (for other conditions), you may suffer more attacks.

Certain kinds of diuretics – loop and thiazide diuretics – are associated with an increased risk of gout. Examples of such diuretics are bendroflumethiazide, furosemide and bumetanide.

Chapter 4

How common is gout and who gets it?

Ask the average person about their perception of gout, and who is most likely to suffer from it, and they'll probably describe a rather portly man, an 18th-century *'Lord Of the Manor'*, drinking claret or port and eating a leg of mutton in his enormous stately home!

But this image of gout being a 'rich man's disease' is exactly that – an image, and one with little or no basis in reality.

The truth in our 21st century world is very different...

- Gout affects about 1 in 200 adults worldwide, with over 1.5 million UK sufferers...

"One in 40 people in the UK is affected, according to analysis of 15 years of results, in the Annals of the Rheumatic Diseases journal." [SOURCE: http://www.bbc.co.uk/news/health-25742467]

- Men are nine times more likely to suffer from gout than women, with a heightened incidence in Asians.

- Gout usually affects men aged 40 years and over, and women over 65 years.

- The incidence of gout increases with age, affecting 7% of men aged over 75 in the UK.

Cases of gout are on the increase because of three major factors:

1. The ageing population

2. The increasing incidence of the metabolic syndrome (more on this in the next paragraph)

3. And changes in our diet (changes which aren't always for the better...)

What is metabolic syndrome? Do you have it? (See for yourself below...)

It's a health condition that features three or more of the following medical symptoms:

- Abdominal [central] obesity, (i.e. a large waist and too big a *'spare tyre'*).

- High blood pressure

- High fasting blood levels of glucose

- High blood levels of triglycerides (a type of fat)

- Low blood levels of high-density cholesterol (HDL), which is the "protective" cholesterol.

Why is metabolic syndrome important, and how does it affect your health?

Having metabolic syndrome increases the risk of developing cardiovascular disease, particularly coronary heart disease, heart failure and type 2 diabetes.

Currently it affects nearly one-third of the population, and is a major risk factor for developing gout.

Is gout associated with any other diseases?

Increasingly, doctors are viewing gout as more than just a joint disease.

Other conditions often associated with it include:

- high blood pressure
- obesity
- osteoarthritis
- diabetes
- high blood levels of fat
- chronic kidney disease
- ischaemic heart disease
- heart failure

It's important you're aware of this, because having other associated medical conditions can limit your pain-relief options, and can also contribute to long-term health complications.

> "Having a gout flareup in your toe is like having your toe catch on fire, and then putting out the fire by slamming it with a hammer."
>
> *Anon*

Chapter 5

What are the symptoms of gout?

Gout is a form of arthritis, which is why it causes pain and discomfort in your joints.

- You'll know when you're having a typical gout attack due to the sudden onset of severe pain, swelling, warmth, and redness of a joint.

- Its diagnosis is almost always obvious to a doctor as, apart from infection, there are very few other conditions with which it may be confused.

- Although any joint can be affected - and sometimes more than one - the most common joint to be affected by gout is the first metatarsophalangeal joint – in plain English, your big toe – when it is sometimes known as *podagra*.

Other fairly common areas for gout attacks are in the feet, ankles, knees, and elbows.

An acute attack of gout typically reaches its peak in 12 to 24 hours, after which time it slowly starts to improve even without treatment. Full recovery typically takes a week or two.

Although acute attacks of gout can occur quite often, typically they occur fairly infrequently, e.g. once or twice a year or even only once or twice in a lifetime.

For some sufferers, gout can be a chronic recurring condition with multiple severe attacks that occur at short intervals, often with no completely pain-free period in between attacks.

This is called chronic gout and can lead to significant joint destruction and deformity – and sometimes may even be confused with other forms of chronic inflammatory arthritis such as rheumatoid arthritis. Often uric acid tophi are present.

NB - For more on this, please refer to *Chapter 2: Are there different types of gout?*

"Some diseases that afflict humans today,
such as malaria, gout and cancer,
are truly ancient
and were handed down to us
from our distant ancestors.
By studying the distribution
of these diseases
in other living and fossil organisms,
we can gain insights
into the nature of these diseases."

Christopher Beard,
curator and specialist in vertebrate paleontology at
Carnegie Museum of Natural History Museum

Chapter 6

How do doctors diagnose gout?
(And how they can relieve your gout pain)

If you go to your doctor with classic symptoms – sudden swelling, redness and severe pain of a big toe, known as *podagra* – the diagnosis is sufficiently obvious that there is no need at that point for further tests or investigations.

But if the symptoms are less typical or involve other joints, the only way to make a definitive diagnosis of gout is to demonstrate the presence of tophi.

- Tophi are monosodium urate crystals in the synovial fluid (the viscous, fluid found in the cavities of synovial joints, which reduces friction between the surfaces of the bones of the joints during movement).

- In order to see whether you have tophi in your joints, your doctor will use a procedure known as joint aspiration – inserting a hollow needle into the joint to sample the crystals and the synovial fluid.

- The procedure is necessary only when symptoms are atypical or involve other joints.

- The procedure may be done either during an acute attack or between attacks (the inter-critical period).

- It also allows a doctor to distinguish between gout and two other conditions:
    - A condition called *pseudogout*, in which the crystals are not of monosodium urate but calcium pyrophosphate; and
    - Septic (infected) arthritis.

How useful are blood tests?

Measuring blood uric acid levels are fairly unimportant in diagnosing gout, but are very important in deciding if the dose of preventive medication is correct.

Contrary to popular belief, treating someone just because he or she has a high uric acid level is not good practice.

Although the risk of clinical gout increases with increasing concentrations of serum uric acid, not everyone with *hyperuricaemia* (high blood levels of uric acid) will develop gout.

There is no evidence to support drug treatment of people with hyperuricaemia but no symptoms of gout.

A patient with confirmed gout may have normal serum uric acid levels, especially during an acute attack, when levels are often reduced: this is because the excretion of uric acid by the kidneys increases during the acute phase.

This doesn't mean that blood tests have no place in the early stages of gout, and it's useful to screen for co-existing medical conditions (see above).

Typically the tests would be for blood levels of urea and electrolytes, glucose, lipids (fats), and estimated glomerular filtration rate (a test that gives an indication of the state of the kidneys).

As well as blood tests, the initial management of a patient with gout will also include measuring and managing high blood pressure, overweight, smoking, alcohol and cardiovascular risk (risk of heart attack and stroke).

X-rays and ultrasound – do you need them to diagnose gout?

X-rays and other imaging are not usually needed to diagnose gout. Plain x-rays are often normal, although x-rays can sometimes be useful to diagnose chronic gout. Currently ultrasound is not routinely used but it is possible that it may prove useful in the future.

Can gout be misdiagnosed?

In a word 'yes', especially if too much emphasis is made on the blood uric acid (UA) level.

Gout can occur at any blood UA level. In addition, during attacks of gout attacks, the blood UA level becomes higher than usual in some gout patients but lower in others.

Roughly half of gout patients have normal UA level during the attacks. This means that the diagnosis of gout based mainly on the blood UA level during a gout attack is unreliable.

<u>As we've seen above, a joint fluid test which visually identifies the MSU crystals in the joint fluid is more accurate in diagnosing gout.</u>

It's important to remember that the diagnosis of gout is not an exact science. The American Rheumatology Association's criteria for diagnosis of acute gout are:

— the presence of MSU crystals in the joint fluid and/or in a tophus, and/or

— the presence of six or more of the following 13 criteria based on clinical, laboratory and x-ray findings:
    • More than one attack of acute arthritis (joint inflammation)
    • Maximum inflammation developed within one day
    • Attack of a single joint
    • Redness over joints
    • Metatarsophalangeal joint (the joint between the foot and the toe itself) of the big toe painful or swollen
    • Attack of the big toe in one foot
    • Attack of heel joint in one foot
    • Tophus, deposits of MSU crystals in tissues (proven or suspected)

- Hyperuricemia (high blood levels of uric acid)
- Asymmetrical swelling within a joint on x-ray
- Subcortical cysts without erosions on x-ray
- MSU crystals in joint fluid during attack
- Joint fluid culture negative for organisms during attack

Are there diseases or conditions which can be mistaken for gout?

There are many conditions that can be confused with gout. These include:

- Microfractures – tiny fractures in a bone caused when the force applied to a bone is greater than the strength of that bone

- Septic Arthritis – an acute and potentially extremely serious infective arthritis

- Reactive Arthritis – a inflammation in one or a few joints caused by infection in another part of the body

- Rhabdomyolysis - a condition in which damaged skeletal muscle tissue breaks down rapidly, causing severe muscle pain

- Psoriatic Arthritis – arthritis associated with psoriasis, a mainly skin condition

- Rheumatoid Arthritis – a severe form of arthritis

- Pseudogout – a condition caused by the accumulation of crystals of calcium pyrophosphate dihydrate in or around a joint, typically the knee joint

- Other Crystal Arthritis, the commonest being apatite crystals which are deposited not only inside joints but in tendons, causing calcific tendinitis

The big danger is if you have hyperuricemia and gout, every time you have a painful inflamed joint, it's automatically diagnosed as gout without much thought as to other possibilities.

The economic cost of gout

"Gout affects an estimated 8 million Americans, among whom those working have an average of almost 5 more absence days annually than workers without gout. On average, the incremental annual cost of care for a gout patient is estimated at over $3,000 compared with a non-gouty individual. Even though comorbidities common in gout patients account for a portion of this increased economic burden, the total annual cost attributable to gout patients in the United States is likely in the tens of billions of dollars and comparable to those of other major chronic disorders, such as migraine and Parkinson's disease."

SOURCE: Current Therapeutic Research, December 2013, Volume 75, Pages 1–4, A Revised Estimate of the Burden of Illness of Gout (Authors: Albert Wertheimer, PhD, MBA, Robert Morlock, PhD, Michael A. Becker, MD)

Chapter 7

What are the possible complications of gout?

On a basic level, gout is a very painful condition. But although the short-term pain might pass fairly quickly, your gout condition can lead to a number of serious long-term health conditions. These include...

Tophi

- As discussed earlier in this book, these are white or yellow lumps of uric acid crystal that form under the skin.

- Although usually painless, they can form in awkward places, such as at the ends of your fingers.

- Tophi usually develop several years after your first attack of gout, but sometimes they can develop even before then.

- They're most commonly found on the toes, heels, knees, forearms, elbows and fingers. Although very rare, they can form in the spinal or even the vocal cords.

- Occasionally tophi become inflamed and can even produce a discharge consisting of a mixture of pus and white toothpaste-like material.

- Sometimes tophi become so large that they can make everyday tasks, such as dressing or preparing food, extremely painful, in which event they may require surgical removal. A joint may become so severely damaged by tophi that it needs to be replaced.

Kidney stones

- Around 10-25% of people with high levels of uric acid form uric acid crystals in their kidneys, resulting in kidney stones.

- As you probably know, kidney stones can interfere with the flow of urine which causes pain on passing urine and the desire to urinate frequently.

- Kidney stones can also cause an infection in the urinary system. Fortunately most kidney stones are small enough to pass through the urinary system on their own, usually within a day or two.

- HEALTH TIP: Drinking plenty of fluids helps to flush out stones, but by this I mean water and NOT alcohol, spirits or soft drinks containing high levels of fructose.

The Psychological effects of gout – how you'll be affected... The severe pain of acute gout can be not only physically but psychologically debilitating, sometimes resulting in anxiety and depression. If this happens, help from your doctor is important.

"A taste for drink, combined with gout,
Had doubled him up forever."

Sir William Schwenck Gilbert

"Some philosophers, and the ancient Stoics among the rest, derived a topic of consolation under all afflictions, while they taught their pupils that those ills under which they laboured were, in reality, goods to the universe; and that to an enlarged view, which could comprehend the whole system of nature, every event became an object of joy and exultation. But though this topic be specious and sublime, it was soon found in practice weak and ineffectual. You would surely irritate than appease a man lying under the racking pains of the gout by preaching up to him the rectitude of those general laws."

David Hume,
An Enquiry Concerning Human Understanding (1748),
VIII: Of Liberty and Necessity, Part II

Part 2

How you can treat your gout pain

You now know what gout is…

In Section 1 of this book, you saw what causes gout…

You also know how to spot the symptoms of gout (and know whether or not you have gout – or another, similar condition…)

But if you know for certain you have gout, and you're suffering its agonising effects, then you want to relieve that pain quickly and effectively.

And that's exactly what you'll get in part 2 of *Goutbusters*, which reveals:

- Suffering a gout attack? Here are the three simple things you can do right away to relieve your pain (page 44).

- The best medication to take for your gout pain (page 45).

- Which combinations of drugs you must NEVER mix when treating your gout (page 46).

- The brand-new breakthrough treatments you can use to treat your gout pain. But how effective are they? See for yourself on page 48…

Please turn over the page…

Chapter 8

ɔw is gout treated?

art 1: Simple measures

1. During a gout attack, it is important to do three things:

   - Rest,

   - Raise your limb, and

   - Avoid accidentally knocking or damaging the affected joint.

2. Keeping the affected joint cool will also help.

   - Remove surrounding clothing and apply an ice pack to it - I suggest a bag of frozen peas or some ice cubes wrapped inside a towel.

3. Apply the ice pack to your joint for approximately 20 minutes.

   - Do not apply ice directly to your skin

   - Do not apply it for more than 20 minutes at a time (because this could damage the skin).

Chapter 9

How is gout treated?

Part 2: Anti-inflammatory painkillers

The aim of treatment in acute gout is to provide rapid pain relief and to reduce swelling.

The first port of call as regards to pain-relieving medication are usually non-steroidal anti-inflammatory drugs, or NSAIDs (e.g. naproxen, diclofenac, indomethacin, etoricoxib) or colchicine – see below for more about this drug.

Naproxen is probably the most widely used drug for treating the effects of gout, since it is fast acting and relatively safe.

That said, you need to be a little bit careful about using it, particularly if you suffer from one of the conditions listed below:

- Ischaemic heart disease
- Heart failure
- Chronic kidney disease
- A history of gastrointestinal ulcers, bleeds, or perforations.

You should continue your treatment until the attack has resolved, which typically takes from one to two weeks.

Chapter 10

How is gout treated?

Part 3: Other drugs

One of the other drugs you can use to treat gout is called colchicine.

- Colchicine is a naturally occurring alkaloid. It was originally extracted from plants of the genus Colchicum (autumn crocus, otherwise known as Colchicum autumnale, or 'meadow saffron').

- Although very effective in the treatment of acute gout, it has the drawback of often producing severe diarrhoea or vomiting, or both.

- This is why it's used less often these days in favour of NSAIDs unless there are contraindications to or intolerance of NSAIDs.

Another drawback to colchicines use is that there are quite a few drugs which – if you're currently taking them for other conditions – might increase its risk of toxicity.

- These include amiodarone, ciclosporin, digoxin, diltiazem, fibrates, Antifungals (e.g. itraconazole, ketoconazole), macrolide antibiotics, protease inhibitors, statins and verapamil.

Colchicine has a very interesting history. The autumn crocus, from which it was originally derived, was used by Egyptian physicians around 1500 BC, an Egyptian medical papyrus.

The first mention of its use in gout was in De Materia Medica by Pedanius Dioscorides in the first century AD.

It was used in Greece around 550 AD, in Persia around 1000 AD, and in France in the sixteenth century. It was used for the first time in London in the early seventeenth century.

The actual drug colchicine was first isolated in 1820 by two French chemists and then purified and given the name colchicine by the German scientists, Geiger and Hesse, in 1833.

Steroid injections can also be useful in the treatment of acute gout.

- Injection into the affected joint can produce rapid and highly effective treatment.

- It is a specialised procedure and is generally carried out only in hospitals or specialist units.

- An alternative is oral steroids in the form of prednisolone, typically at a dose of around 30 mg a day for five days, and this is probably as effective as NSAIDs.

"Pain, scorned by yonder gout-ridden wretch, endured by yonder dyspeptic in the midst of his dainties, borne bravely by the girl in travail. Slight thou art, if I can bear thee, short thou art if I cannot bear thee!"

Seneca, (Roman philosopher, mid-1st century AD)

Chapter 11

How is gout treated?

Part 4: Very new and emerging treatments

As well as the simple and conventional ways available for you to treat your gout, there are also plenty of alternative, new treatments you can use.

The first of these is a drug already used to treat rheumatoid arthritis, Anakinra.

- Anakinra is an interleukin-1 (IL-1) receptor antagonist. It blocks the biologic activity of naturally occurring IL-1, including inflammation.

- Studies suggest that Anakinra is effective, relatively well tolerated with short-term use, and could be a good alternative for treating gouty arthritis in patients for whom conventional therapies are ineffective or contraindicated. However Its long-term use could be limited by infectious complications.

The second treatment is Canakinumab.

- This is a fully human monoclonal anti-interleukin (IL)-1β antibody that selectively blocks IL-1β.

- It has been found to be superior to colchicine in treating gout attacks, both in terms of reducing pain and the risk of new gout attacks.

- Canakinumab's long half-life contributes to its prolonged anti-inflammatory effects.

And there's also Rilonacept, an interleukin-1 inhibitor.

- Studies have shown that Rilonacept markedly reduces the occurrence of gout flares (when people that are prone to gout suddenly suffer the symptoms of the disease) associated with the initiation of uric acid lowering therapy (ULT).

- The efficacy and safety profile suggests that Rilonacept may have the potential to improve long-term disease control for some patients;.

- It does this by improving adherence to ULT by reducing flares during the first months after ULT initiation.

****

Other advances in genome technology are helping to increase doctors' understanding of uric acid metabolism, and are likely to lead to further new therapies.

As well as medication, there's another key factor you need to take into account if you want to stop gout from killing you, and that's... *Please turn over the page to find out what it is...*

"A man can no more separate age and covetousness than a' can part young limbs and lechery: but the gout galls the one, and the pox pinches the other; and so both the degrees prevent my curses. Boy! [...]
I can get no remedy against this consumption of the purse: borrowing only lingers and lingers it out, but the disease is incurable. [...]
A pox of this gout! or, a gout of this pox! for the one or the other plays the rogue with my great toe."

Shakespeare's Falstaff, Henry IV Part 1

Part 3

How to manage your gout pain (and get rid of it fast)

In this section, you'll discover...

- The simple ways for you to prevent gout attacks (easier than you might think! Find the *'need to know'* facts on page 53...).

- Suffering regular gout attacks? Here are the medical drugs to take (and the best times to take them for maximum pain relief (pages 55-56).

- What to do if you can't take – or are allergic to – conventional drugs (pages 58-59).

- The common fruit you can eat to keep gout attacks at bay (page 62)

- The truth about Vitamin C and gout (does it prevent attacks? The medical facts uncovered on page 62).

- Can you really relieve your gout pain with alternative and complementary medicine? (answers on pages 63-64)

- The 15 'diet do's and don'ts': what to eat – and what not to eat – to stop and prevent your agonising gout attacks – (pages 66-69)

- Supplements – are they good or bad for gout? (page 70)

- Herbs – do the positives outweigh the negatives? (See our controversial findings for yourself on page 72)

- Homeopathy – the facts and the fiction (INCLUDES: the 'external' therapies and treatments you can use to reduce the painful effects of gout – page 75).

- Two things you should do in order to manage your gout (details on page 79).

- Future research — what's being done to relieve your pain? (page 80)

- CASE STUDY #1: how John overcame his gout (and the simple treatment which helped to end his crippling attacks — page 82).

- CASE STUDY #2: how Nick Wrathall, editor, *Goutbusters*, overcame his gout... (page 84)

- **Dr Spira's *Gout Traffic-Light Test*** (which foods can you eat without fear? Which ones can you eat in moderation? And which ones should you avoid eating where at all possible? All is revealed on pages 87-94)

- Why good girls don't get gout (if you're a woman sufferer, here are the *'need to know'* facts — page 95), *and much, much more...*

Chapter 12

How can I prevent further gout attacks?

Part 1: Lifestyle

FACT: you can take all the best drugs in the world, but if your lifestyle and diet are poor, then the gout medication will not work.

So it's important to take into account that non-drug management of gout is all about modifying risk factors, including lifestyle.

A key feature of this is DIET...

This means that your diet should be focused on reducing the intake of purine-rich foods, such as red meat and seafood, and alcohol, especially beer.

For overweight patients, losing weight is very useful.

The combination of diet and weight loss has a moderate but significant effect on reducing uric acid levels and lowering the frequency of gout attacks.

Other aspects of diet that may be helpful include increasing your consumption of:

- Dairy products
- Vitamin C
- Coffee
- Cherries

...and reducing your consumption of fructose and sugar-sweetened soft drinks.

If you're overweight, the levels of uric acid in your blood are likely to rise, and losing weight is likely to help reduce uric acid levels.

- The best way to lose weight is by following a balanced, calorie-controlled diet.

- Crash diets are bad.

- A high-protein, low-carbohydrate diet should be avoided because high-protein foods often contain high levels of purines.

Regular exercise can also be very helpful for reducing both the intensity and frequency of gout attacks

- Apart from its general health benefits, exercise lowers blood urate levels and decreases the risk of developing gout.

- Of course, it's important to avoid exercise that puts strain on the affected muscles or joints. Swimming is a good way to stay fit without putting pressure on joints.

Chapter 13

How can I prevent further gout attacks?

Part 2: Prescribed medicines

Like most gout sufferers, you'll probably be familiar with the drug, allopurinol, which is used to lower blood levels of uric acid.

Allopurinol, which has several different brand names, the commonest in the UK being Zyloric, is what is known as a *'purine analog'* and inhibits the action in the body of an enzyme called xanthine oxidase.

Xanthine oxidase is essential for the oxidation of two chemicals in the body called xanthine and hypoxanthine, a process that results in the production of uric acid.

The big question is *if* and *when* you should start using allopurinol.

- Most doctors advise its use in patients with recurrent acute gout, chronic gout or tophi, x-ray damage to joints, kidney failure, or the formation of stones made of uric acid.

- But not all of them agree at what point allopurinol should be prescribed in recurrent acute attacks of gout.

- Some doctors advise you to start using allopurinol after the first attack, when the amount of crystal in the joint(s) is small, and there hasn't been any significant joint damage.

- Other doctors advise waiting until two or more attacks have occurred within a year.

- Given that a recurrence of attacks is common, most doctors will discuss treatment options with you early on.

The commonest time to start allopurinol is around two to four weeks after an acute attack of gout has resolved.

If you start using the drug too soon, there's a risk it might actually make your attack worse.

What's more, it's easier for you to take in the information about whether or not to start a drug when your mind isn't clouded by pain.

It's also important to remember that starting to use allopurinol is generally a lifelong commitment.

- Allopurinol is started at low dose, typically 100 mg daily, and is increased in 100 mg increments every few weeks until the blood level of uric acid is below 360 µmol/L.

- This has been found to be the highest optimal level in order to stop further acute attacks, help tophi to disappear, and reduce the amount of crystals in the joint(s).

- Some doctors suggest reducing uric acid to below 300 µmol/L, at least for the year or two, as this seems to accelerate the rate of elimination of tophi and crystals.

For many patients, a typical effective dose would be around 400-500 mg a day.

- The maximum dose is 900 mg per day, although such a high dose is rarely necessary.

- During the period that the dose is being adjusted upwards, monthly blood tests are necessary – this is to monitor the blood cells, kidney and liver function, and uric acid levels.

- Incidentally, because allopurinol is excreted through the kidneys, if you suffer from kidney failure and patients taking diuretics are given lower doses and increases are done more slowly.

- This is because of the risk of the rare but potentially life threatening allopurinol hypersensitivity syndrome – which involves severe skin reactions and kidney and liver dysfunction.

The good news is that 90% of patients are able to take allopurinol without problems.

- IMPORTANT: since the drug partially dissolves crystals, which results in increased shedding of crystals, you may experience an acute attack of gout when they start taking the drug.

- This is why – if you're taking allopurinol – you need to make sure the dose has to be increased gradually (and not all in one go).

- In addition, a low dose of an NSAID in colchicines is sometimes also prescribed up to six months until a stable dose of allopurinol has been reached.

- Once you're on allopurinol, don't stop using it if you have an acute gout attack.

*"Supposing I'm intolerant of allopurinol.
Are there any alternatives?"*

The main alternative is a drug called febuxostat, a drug you''ll find out more about (together with other similar drugs) in the next chapter. Treatment with allopurinol is lifelong.

Once the dose has been stabilised, blood tests are usually done every six months to monitor treatment. Once the gout crystals have been cleared and there are no more attacks, you can adjust the dose of allopurinol to maintain uric acid levels of around 300-360 µmol/L, and at this stage blood test monitoring need be done only annually or even every two years.

Chapter 14

How can I prevent further gout attacks?

Part 3: Other prescribed medicines

The main alternative to allopurinol is a drug called febuxostat which is recommended for use when allopurinol cannot be taken.

- Technically it is a type of drug known as a *non-purine xanthine oxidase inhibitor*.

- Although perhaps not quite so effective as allopurinol at reducing uric acid levels, it has the advantage that it's metabolised mainly by the liver.

- In practical terms, this means you don't need dose reduction in mild or moderate kidney failure, and it doesn't interact with the blood-thinning drug, warfarin.

However, it isn't recommended for use if you suffer from ischaemic heart disease or heart failure, or if you've received an organ transplant.

NOTE: to try to reduce the frequency and severity of this side-effect, your doctor may prescribe you regular daily oral NSAID or colchicine for up to six months following the start of febuxostat as prophylaxis preventative treatment.

Common side effects of febuxostat include:

- An increased number of acute gout attacks
- Diarrhoea
- Nausea
- Headaches
- Skin rashes

More serious symptoms include breathing difficulties and facial swelling, and these usually necessitate stopping the drug.

Febuxostat is not suitable for people with heart problems or serious kidney disease.

- It's difficult for you to lower uric acid levels if, for whatever reason, you cannot take allopurinol and febuxostat.

- There are other drugs, such as sulfinpyrazone, probenecid and benzbromarone, but these are not widely available.

- Sulphinpyrazone and probenecid are not as effective as other types of uric acid lowering drugs and are not suitable if you suffer from kidney disease.

- Benzbromarone is more effective in removing uric acid, and can be used if you have kidney disease.

Chapter 15

How can I prevent further gout attacks?

Part 4: Vitamin C

- The flavonoids are a group of plant pigments largely responsible for the colours of fruits and flowers. In addition, they also help protect plants against environmental stress.

- In humans, flavonoids modify the reaction to allergens (those are the substances that produce an abnormally vigorous immune response, in which the immune system fights off what it sees as a threat that would otherwise be harmless to the body), and infectious agents such as bacteria and viruses.

- Flavonoids also have anti-inflammatory properties.

- <u>Perhaps the most important flavonoids for people with various forms of arthritis, including gout, are those that provide the colours of blackberries, blueberries, cherries and grapes.</u>

- Some of their properties include:
  - The ability to increase vitamin C levels within our bodies' cells
  - Decreasing the leakiness and breakage of tiny blood vessels
  - Protecting your body against free radical damage – more about free radicals in a moment.

In addition, flavonoids inhibit enzymes secreted by our white blood cells that would otherwise destroy collagen structures during inflammation.

- Eating around 250 g of fresh cherries each day has been shown to be effective in lowering uric acid levels and preventing attacks of gout.

What are free radicals?

Free radicals are molecules with unpaired electrons which are constantly looking for another electron. As a result, they are very reactive and cause damage to surrounding molecules, that can cause a great deal of harm to your body.

Free radicals are everywhere - in the air, in our bodies, in things around us. They are the reason, for example, that plastics deteriorate and paint fades.

More important for you and your health, they cause ageing-related illnesses and can contribute to heart attacks, stroke and cancers.

The good news is that antioxidants, including flavonoids contained in dark berries, help to prevent or reduce free radical damage.

Is there scientific evidence that vitamin C helps prevent gout?

- A 2009 study showed that vitamin C can reduce the risk of developing gout.

- In the study, 46,994 men were followed up over several years. Compared with men with a vitamin C intake of less than 250 mg a day, those that took 1,000-1,499 mg per day had a 34% lower risk of gout, and those who took 1,500 mg per day had a 45% lower risk of gout.

- The study suggests that taking vitamin C supplements may help prevent gout, but not all doctors agree with the findings. Other studies in healthy volunteers suggest that vitamin C supplements reduce blood uric acid levels.

However another very recent piece of research contradicted the findings.

Doctors in New Zealand recruited 40 gout patients who had blood uric acid levels greater than the treatment target level of 0.36mmol.

20 patients taking allopurinol were given an additional 500 mg dose of vitamin C daily or had the dose of allopurinol increased, while the other 20 patients were either started on allopurinol or 500 mg of vitamin C daily.

The study showed that a modest vitamin C dose for eight weeks did not lower uric acid levels to a clinically significant degree in gout patients, but did increase blood levels of vitamin C.

How might vitamin C work in helping to reduce the risk of gout?

If vitamin C does help – and that's a big 'if' – it's likely that it increases the excretion of uric acid in the urine.

Again, we don't know the exact mechanism but it's probably to do with the way the kidneys excrete uric acid. It's possible too that vitamin C may also reduce production of uric acid.

So how might cherries help gout sufferers?

Cherries have been reported to lower uric acid levels in women, and they have also been reported to reduce the number of gout attacks. How they might do this is not clear.

One possibility is that cherries increase uric acid excretion via the kidneys and may lower uric acid production.

There are also other anti-inflammatory chemicals in cherries that may have an effect, which means the amount of vitamin C in cherries is probably not high enough to have any effect.

So the jury is out on whether vitamin C has a beneficial effect on treating gout...

Chapter 16

Alternative & Complementary medicine

As well as medication, diet and lifestyle (and the newer, cutting-edge drugs available), there are plenty of other ways you can tackle and overcome your gout pain.

For many people, alternative and complementary medicines provide other solutions, some of which are discussed below, the first one being...

Acupuncture – can it really relieve gout pain?

Recently published research suggests that acupuncture is an effective complementary treatment for patients with gout.

- Researchers at Kyung Hee University in Seoul, South Korean, analysed the results of ten different English and Chinese randomised controlled trials involving 852 gout patients.

- All the trials involved acupuncture in combination with conventional gout therapy.

- Six studies, involving 512 patients, pointed strongly to a reduction in uric acid levels in gout patients who had received complementary acupuncture treatment as compared to the control group.

- However a further two studies, involving 120 patients, showed no significant difference.

- Four further studies, involving 380 patients, suggested a significant decline in the visual signs of gout among members of the treatment group.

SUMMARY: the researchers concluded that acupuncture is effective when combined with traditional gout treatments.

What about other alternative/complementary therapies?

There is a vast range of such therapies.

Although there isn't a lot of hard scientific evidence for their efficacy there's a lot of anecdotal evidence – evidence that comes from the experience of individual patients.

<u>Now whilst this is clearly not as good as scientific evidence, it shouldn't be dismissed.</u>

<u>This is for one simple reason...</u> Much of complementary medicine is to do with substances which are not patented and therefore are not in pharmaceutical companies' interests to research which would be prohibitively expensive.

Preparations made from the secondary tubers of Devil's claw (Harpagophytum procumbens) have been successfully used in patients with rheumatic diseases.

There is some evidence that the ayurvedic Taila (oil) and Ghrita (ghee) prepared with Guduchi (Tinospora cordifolia) may be helpful in gout.

A word of caution: Herbs and supplements that may be helpful for some people may be harmful for others. It's always advisable to consult your doctor before embarking on such therapies.

Blood-letting

Now before you throw your hands up in horror(!), blood-letting can be a good way to treat your gout.

This is because several researchers have suggested a link between uric acid and iron.

- Studies suggests that an alternative treatment for gout may be simply reducing the amount of iron in the body.

- For example, Dr F S Facchini of the University of California, San Francisco, demonstrated the benefit of drawing blood in 12 gout patients, and his findings were published in the highly respected medical journal, Rheumatology (Oxford) in 2003.

- His goal was to investigate whether or not iron removal would improve the outcome of gouty arthritis in humans.

- He aimed to lower iron levels, but not to the point of anaemia – a level referred to as near-iron deficiency, or NID. 12 gout patients had blood removed until they were almost deficient in iron.

- At this level, the subjects had just enough iron to maintain normal red blood cell production, i.e. near-deficiency.

- The patients were monitored for 28 months, and suffered no ill effects from the loss of blood.

- However, they gained significant improvement in their gout. 58% of subjects achieved complete remission from gout attacks, whilst the remainder experienced fewer and less severe attacks.

- Admittedly the sample size of this study was fairly small, but it did point strongly towards the view that reducing iron is an effective alternative treatment for gout.

SUMMARY: a follow-on to this finding is that, if frequent blood donations are not an option, then <u>reducing the amount of available iron in the body through diet is an obvious alternative.</u>

Diet – and the crucial role it plays in getting rid of your gout

We'll look at diet in greater detail later in this book.

However, in this chapter, we'll look at typical dietary advice given by some complementary or alternative therapists, which is much stricter than that given by more conventional health professionals.

How effective this kind of strict advice is difficult to say since the evidence is mainly anecdotal rather than scientific:

Therefore, please find below a brief list of "diet 'do's' and 'don'ts'", which you may find useful to follow...

1. Eat antioxidant foods – these include:

*   Fruits (such as blueberries, cherries, tomatoes)
*   Vegetables (such as bell peppers and squash)

2. Avoid refined foods, including:

*   Pastas
*   Sugar
*   White breads

3. Avoid sugar sweetened soft drinks.

*   This is not a moral lecture, but my editor tells me that he uses bottles of sweetened soft drinks to unblock his drains, as they work better than anything else! So imagine how much harm they do to your body...

4. Cut back on fructose.

5. Eat less red meat

6. Instead of red meat, you should focus on eating the following alternative protein sources, which are all excellent sources of protein:

- Fish
- Soy and beans
- Tofu

7. You should also eat more high fibre foods, such as:

- Oats
- Psyllium seed
- Root vegetables (such as potatoes and yams)

8. Cut out foods that are potential allergens, such as:

- Corn
- Dairy
- Food additives
- Preservatives
- Wheat/gluten

9. Cut down on foods containing oxalates (substances found in plants, animals, and in humans. In chemical terms, oxalates belong to a group of molecules called organic acids).

Oxalate-rich foods include:

- Beans
- Beets
- Black tea
- Chocolate
- Nuts
- Rhubarb
- Spinach
- Strawberries
- Wheat bran

10. Eat foods rich in magnesium and low in calcium:

- Avocado
- Banana
- Barley
- Bran
- Brown rice
- Corn
- Oats
- Potato
- Rye
- Soy

11. Cut down on foods high in purines:

- Anchovies
- Beef
- Goose
- Herring
- Liver
- Kidneys
- Mackerel
- Mussels
- Sweetbreads
- Yeast

Foods with moderate amounts of purines include:

- Asparagus
- Beans
- Dried peas
- Lentils
- Mushrooms
- Other fish (such as shellfish)
- Other meats (such as poultry)
- Shellfish
- Spinach

12. Use healthy cooking oils (such as olive oil or coconut oil).

13. Avoid foods containing trans fatty acids. These are found in commercially baked foods such as:

- Biscuits
- Cakes
- Crackers
- Doughnuts
- Many processed foods
- Margarine
- Onion rings

14. Avoid alcohol.

15. Drink eight glasses of water (bottled or tap – it doesn't matter which) each day.

Whilst this advice has recently been challenged as an essential health regime for everyone, the advice nevertheless holds good, to help you flush uric acid from the body. Always avoid becoming dehydrated.

****

On the next page, you'll find out about one of the most controversial areas of gout management

Supplements - good or bad for gout?

As with diet advice in the previous section, complementary therapists' advice on the use of supplements relies almost entirely on anecdotal rather than scientific evidence.

This is not to say that the advice is wrong, but simply that it hasn't been subject to rigorous scrutiny.

Here are some examples:

– A daily multivitamin.
  - This should contain vitamins A, C, E and B-complex as well as trace minerals such as magnesium, calcium, zinc and selenium.
  - This is to provide antioxidants.
  - Some therapists also advocate higher doses of vitamin C, typically 500-1,000 mg daily.

– Omega-3 fish oils.
  - These are to help decrease inflammation and promote general health.
  - But if you're taking blood thinning medications, such as aspirin or warfarin, you should first consult your doctor.

– N-acetyl cysteine (with a suggestion to take 200 mg daily), as this is another antioxidant.

– IP-6 (inositol hexophosphonate).
  - Check with your alternative health care provider for proper dosing.
  - But, as with omega-3 oils, if you are taking blood thinning medications, such as aspirin or warfarin, you should first consult your doctor.

- Methylsulfonylmethane (MSM)
    - A suggested dose of 3,000 mg twice daily.
    - This is said to help decrease inflammation.

****

On the next page, I discuss another controversial area of gout care, which is not free of unwanted side effects, but can be a very good way to strengthen your body and fight against gout pain.

Full details on the next page...

Herbs – do the positives outweigh the negatives?

The usefulness of herbs in the fight against gout pain is another controversial area.

As with the other complementary treatments I've discussed, there's a good deal of anecdotal evidence that they help some people, but always check first with your doctor.

This is because herbs are not as free of unwanted side effects as you might think. In fact, some can interact with prescribed medications, especially blood thinning medications, such as aspirin or warfarin.

According to complementary therapists, herbs are believed to be useful for strengthening and toning the body's systems.

- They may be in the form of dried extracts (capsules, powders, teas), glycerites (glycerine extracts), or tinctures (alcohol extracts).

- Teas are usually made with 5g (1 teaspoon) of herbs in a cup of hot water, then steep covered for 5-10 minutes for leaves or flowers or 10-20 minutes for roots.

- The usual advice is to drink two to four cups a day.

Typical herbs and similar preparations are:

- Cat's claw (Uncaria tomentosa) is supposed to be good for inflammation and the body's immune system.
    - It also has supposed antibacterial and antifungal properties.
    - Potentially it may worsen some medical conditions such as leukaemia and some autoimmune disorders.
    - Again, as with many herbs, it can interact with prescribed medications, so always check first with your doctor.

- Devil's claw (Harpagophytum procumbens) is advised for pain and inflammation.
  - It can interact with prescribed medications, especially blood thinning medications, such as aspirin or warfarin, so first consult your doctor if you are on these prescribed medications.

- Green tea (Camelia sinensis)
  - This is an antioxidant and is said to be good for the body's immune system.

- Cranberry (Vaccinium macrocarpon).
  - 250 to 500 ml a day of unsweetened cranberry juice is said to be good for the kidneys.

- Bromelain (Ananus comosus) is said to be good for pain and inflammation.
  - Again, it can interact with prescribed medications, especially blood thinning medications, such as aspirin or warfarin, so first consult your doctor if you are on these prescribed medications.

- Turmeric (Curcuma longa) is advised for inflammation.
  - And again, it can interact with prescribed medications, especially blood thinning medications, such as aspirin or warfarin, so first consult your doctor if you are on these prescribed medications.

****

Over the last few chapters, I've spoken to you about the so-called 'ingestibles' (foods, herbs and supplements which you can 'ingest' [swallow]) and how they can affect your gout positively – and negatively.

But they're not the only treatments you can use in the fight against gout.

And over the next few pages, I'll be talking about 'external' therapies and treatments you might decide to use, to reduce the painful effects of gout.

What exactly do I mean by 'external' therapies and treatment?

Find out on the next page…

"In the career of glory one gains many things; the gout and medals, a pension and rheumatism….And also frozen feet, an arm or leg the less, a bullet lodged between two bones which the surgeon cannot extract…. all of these fatigues experienced in your youth, you pay for when you grow old. Because one has suffered in years gone by, it is necessary to suffer more, which does not seem exactly fair."

Elzear Blaze, La Vie Militaire

Homeopathy – the facts and the fiction...

Although there is precious little scientific evidence for its effectiveness, homeopathy has a vast loyal following even amongst many conventional doctors.

And gout is an area which is very popular in this form of therapy.

There are many different homeopathic remedies available to you, and, before choosing the appropriate one for a particular patient, the therapist will take into account your constitutional type including your physical, emotional and psychological makeup.

Typical homeopathic remedies include:

− Belladonna - for hot, painful joints

− Rhus toxicodendron - for swollen joints that are stiff, hot and painful, especially if the pain is worse with cold applications and better with heat

− Ledum – for painful, swollen joints, especially if the pain is worse with heat and better with cold applications

− Aconite - for painful and swollen joints

− Colchicum - for joint pain that is associated with changes in the weather. Also useful if nausea is present during attacks

− Berberis vulgaris - for painful twinges in joints and for kidney stones (which are often associated with gout)

− Bryonia - for painful joints that are better with heat and pressure

Massage therapy

- Massage therapy, using massage oils, can be healing as well as very soothing.

- It's designed to stimulate your metabolism, and improve the circulation of blood to the diseased joints and to the surrounding muscles. The result is to reduce pain and prevent spasms.

Acupressure

- This is a cross between acupuncture and massage therapy.

- Instead of needles, therapists use their palms, fingertips and thumbs to perform deep massage in firm but smooth movements on specific pressure points on the body. Unlike massage therapy, no oils are used.

How effective is massage for relieving gout pain?

When a person has a painful joint (especially when this is a situation that persists for long time), the muscles surrounding the joint begin to tighten in order to stabilise this weak spot.

Posture and movements then adapt to reduce short-term pain, but these adaptations are usually not efficient or pain-free themselves.

According to the US National Center for Complementary and Alternative Medicine (NCCAM), which is part of the National Institutes of Health, massage is one of the most popular complementary therapies.

Why and how massage helps in arthritis is not fully understood but recent research suggests that massage can affect the body's production of certain hormones that are linked to blood pressure, heart rate and other key signs as well as anxiety.

But how safe and effective is massage therapy?

- According to the Touch Research Institute at the University of Miami School of Medicine, which has conducted a good deal of research into the benefits of massage, including in various forms of arthritis such as gout, regular massage of muscles and joints can lead to a significant reduction in pain.

- The Institute has shown that regular massage therapy can lead to improvements in pain, stiffness, movement and overall function of joints.

- A 2006 study from the Touch Research Institute was carried out on 22 adults, mostly women, who had arthritis of the hand or wrist.

- Each patient received four weekly massages and was also taught to massage their sore joints daily at home.

- <u>Just a 15 minute, moderate pressure massage each day led to reduced pain and anxiety and to increased grip strength.</u>

Another highly respected establishment, the University of Medicine and Dentistry of New Jersey, published research (also in 2006).

- Their study examined 68 adults with osteoarthritis of the knee which also happens to be a joint not uncommonly affected by gout.

- The patients were split into two groups –
  - a treatment group and
  - a control group.

- Those in the treatment group received twice-weekly Swedish massage therapy during weeks 1 to 4 and once-weekly massage sessions during weeks 5 to 8.

- The control group received what was described as delayed intervention.

<u>The results of the study were that there was significantly reduced pain and significantly improved functionality of the knee in the treatment group.</u>

SUMMARY: the conclusion of the researchers was that massage therapy seemed to be effective in the treatment of arthritis of the knee.

While, at present, there are no cures for gout, massage can certainly help to control the symptoms of gout, and help you to maintain a normal lifestyle whenever you experience an acute attack of gout.

"For God's sake, hold your tongue, and let me love,
Or chide my palsy, or my gout,
My five grey hairs, or ruined fortune flout, With
wealth your state, your mind with arts improve,
Take you a course, get you a place,
Observe his honour, or his grace,
Or the King's real, or his stamped face
Contemplate; what you will, approve,
So you will let me love."

John Donne

Chapter 17

What is the outlook for me with gout?

You've now seen plenty of ways you can understand, tackle and overcome your painful gout conditions.

But it's important to take into account that further attacks may occur, especially within the first year.

However, with early treatment the outlook is very good. Sometimes attacks become more frequent and affect more joints with joint damage and chronic pain.

With this in mind, I advise two things you should do in order to manage your gout:

1. Trust in a good doctor

2. Read up as much as you can about the condition, but only from reliable sources such as this book and the references discussed later in this book.

These days, gout is a very manageable and controllable condition.

Chapter 18

Future research –
what's being done to relieve your pain?

If you've endured the agony of gout for any amount of time, or you've just found out you suffer from it, you'll have seen in *Goutbusters* that there are plenty of ways both to get rid of it (if you have an attack) AND to prevent it (if you know you have it).

Having said that, there remain many unanswered questions about gout and its treatment.

A recent review of the condition in the *British Medical Journal* identified the following areas for research:

1. Are the risks of heart and arterial disease and kidney disease reduced by lowering blood uric acid levels in people with gout?

2. Which is the most effective and safest treatment for acute gout - a non-steroidal anti-inflammatory drug (NSAID) or colchicine at low doses?

3. How effective are dietary changes and weight loss at lowering blood uric acid levels and treating gout?

4. How effective is stopping diuretics at lowering blood uric acid levels and treating gout?

5. When starting a drug to lower uric acid levels, such as allopurinol that can be slowly increased from a low dose, is it necessary to prevent acute attacks with another drug such as a non-steroidal anti-inflammatory drug (NSAID) or colchicine?

6. When starting medication to lower uric acid levels, what should be the target level of blood uric acid to aim for?

As yet, we do not have the answers to these questions, but progress is being made on a daily basis. And with this book you'll be that much closer to finding effective methods for treating your gout for the rest of your life.

Something that one of my patients found out for himself, and which you can read and learn from as you plan the best ways to manage your gout.

See the full story on the next page...

"How many of our virtues originate in the fear of Death & that while we flatter ourselves that we are melting in Christian Sensibility over the sorrows of our human Brethren and Sisteren, we are in fact, tho' perhaps unconsciously, moved at the prospect of our own End for who sincerely pities Sea-sickness, Toothache, or a fit of the Gout in a lusty Good-liver of 50?"

Samuel Taylor Coleridge

Chapter 19

Case study #1: how John overcame his gout...

Like many people with this painful condition, the first gout attack came as a nasty shock.

At the age of 53, John* (not his real name) suddenly woke up one night with severe pain in his right big toe (*podagra*).

He called his GP who sent him to hospital where he was diagnosed with acute gout. He was prescribed an anti-inflammatory painkiller but no other treatment.

John read up about gout and was concerned about the long-term outlook.

Because he was wary of taking long-term medication, he asked his GP if he could control his gout by watching his diet.

His GP agreed and prescribed further anti-inflammatory drugs to have to hand if John experienced another acute attack.

John stuck to his diet but unfortunately – in spite of his new and improved diet - he had recurrent attacks of gout.

These were always extremely painful and meant he couldn't drive, so couldn't go to work. Eventually he realised that diet alone wasn't the answer.

He went back to his GP who took a blood test which showed his uric acid level to be 574 µmol/L. This was high, so the doctor started him on a low dose of allopurinol (200 mg).

John still continued to get attacks, so his GP increased the dose to 300 mg.

A month later a further blood test revealed his uric acid to have fallen dramatically to 268 µmol/L – within the normal range.

Since then John has remained on the allopurinol and has had no further attacks. His only regret is that he didn't start on allopurinol sooner.

"The General has got the gout,
and Mrs. Maitland the jaundice.
Miss Debary, Susan, and Sally, all in black,
but without any stature,
made their appearance,
and I was as civil to them
as their bad breath would allow me."

Jane Austen

Case study #2: how Nick Wrathall, Editor, *Goutbusters*, overcame his gout...

NOTE: Nick Wrathall is not a doctor or scientific expert so this does not, as such, constitute any kind of medical evidence. Instead it's a brief description – in layman's terms - of the tools and strategies he used to bring his gout under control, and make it a distant memory. The words which follow are Nick's...

****

Since my first-ever gout attack at the age of 38, I've left no stone unturned in my search for simple, safe and effective ways to relieve gout pain when it strikes, and also to prevent attacks from happening in the first place.

Whilst I'm no doctor – and what works for me, may not work for you - I've been fortunate enough to cut my gout attacks to almost zero, even when the top of my big toe starts aching (the classic *'canary in the coalmine'* signal that a gout attack could be on the way).

So here's how I've managed my gout attacks over the last few years (PLEASE NOTE: this does not in any way constitute medical advice, so if symptoms persist, please contact your doctor)...

1. Cherry concentrate – one of the first things Dr Spira suggested I used was drinking a cherry concentrate solution. Just ask at your local health food shop and they'll be able to recommend a suitable brand for you.

2. Barley Grass Powder – I think we tend to eat a lot of food which is too acidic, and can lead to gout attacks. One way I've found of combatting this is to drink a glass of barley grass powder twice a day, once in the morning and once last thing at night. It also helps with digestion.

3. Cutting out sugar from my diet – when it comes to gout, you've seen what Dr Spira has said about sugary drinks and their potential for causing gout attacks.

   Anecdotal evidence also suggests that sugar is more addictive than crack cocaine! I should know – I used to have a very sweet tooth, and knew the price and quality of every type of chocolate around.

   But sugary treats cost you, in your wallet and your body, and sugar seems to be in everything – chocolate, drinks, sauces, even certain types of chicken!

   Going 'cold turkey' is tough at first (I had splitting headaches and sweats), but it's well worth it, and since cutting sugar out of my diet, my gout attacks have decreased significantly, both in number and intensity.

4. Cut down on food portion sizes – not only will this lower the risk of gout (and other diseases and conditions linked to being overweight), it will also save you a lot of money from your weekly shopping bill.

   My suggestion is to cut out all sugary foods (see point 3 above), and increase the amount of fruit and vegetables (particularly green leafy ones) you eat.

5. Proper rest and sleep – again, anecdotal evidence, but I've found that my gout attacks are often triggered when I'm not getting enough sleep. Perhaps you have found this too? On the positive side, I can't remember ever having any gout attack when I'd been sleeping properly.

6. More exercise – another good way to keep gout at bay is movement. Even if it's something as simple as walking or cycling, I think it's vital you start and continue some form of exercise, together with a weight-loss programme. Speaking of which...

7. Losing weight – like a lot of people, my work involves sitting down for most of the day. And also like a lot of people, weight gain is a gradual process which occurs over many years, until you receive a wake-up call.

   Mine was seeing myself presenting a marketing conference, and being horrified at how fat I was. Maybe you have this realisation when you're struggling to put on trousers, or a young relative says, "You're fat!" (or something similar).

That *'video nasty'* was mine…

As luck would have it, a new gym opened down the road from me, which I joined and exercise in regularly, and this has helped me to lose 35 pounds (15.91 Kgs).

"The rich ate and drank freely,
accepting gout and apoplexy
as things that ran mysteriously
in respectable families."

George Eliot

Chapter 20

Various foods, their purine content and what can make your gout worse – The 'Traffic Light' Test

In Chapter 3 of *Goutbusters*, I told you about purines, and how two-thirds of uric acid comes from the breakdown of purines in our bodies, whilst around one-third come from purines in our food.

With this in mind, and to help you make the best food choices to manage your symptoms of gout, I've put together a 'traffic light' list of foods.

This is to show you which foods contain high, medium and low amounts of purines, in other words, the ones to avoid eating where at all possible, the ones you can eat in moderation, and the ones you can eat without fear.

HIGH PURITINE CONTENT 'Red' Foods	Total purines mg uric acid / 100 mg food (typical values)
Yeast, Brewer's	1810
Neck sweetbread, calf's	1260
Yeast, Baker's	680
Ox liver	554
Pig's heart	530
Pig's liver	515
Mushroom, flat, edible Boletus, dried	488
Fish, sardines in oil	480
Calf's liver	460
Ox spleen	444

MODERATE PURITINE CONTENT 'Amber' Foods	Total purines mg uric acid / 100 mg food (typical values)
Fish, sardine, pilchard	345
Pig's kidney	334
Fish, trout	297
Fish, Tuna in oil	290
Ox kidney	269
Fish, Tuna	257
Ox heart	256
Chicken's liver	243
Fish, Redfish (ocean perch)	241
Sheep's heart	241
Fish, Anchovy	239
Black gram (mungo bean), seed, dry	222
Fish, Herring, Matje cured	219
Calf's kidney	218
Fish, Herring, Atlantic	210
Bean, Soya, seed, dry	190
Fish, Herring roe	190
Lamb (muscles only)	182
Fish, Halibut	178
Chicken (breast with skin)	175
Veal, muscles only	172
Fish, salmon	170
Poppy seed, dry	170
Pork muscles only	166
Goose	165
Sausage, liver (liverwurst)	165
Fish, Carp	160

Ox tongue	160
Pork leg (hind leg)	160
Chicken, boiling fowl, average	159
Pork fillet	150
Pork shoulder with skin (blade of shoulder)	150
Turkey, young animal, average, with skin	150
Veal, knuckle with bone	150
Veal, leg of veal with bone	150
Veal, neck with bone	150
Shrimp, brown	147
Fish, Mackerel	145
Pork chop with bone	145
Caviar	144
Sunflower seed, dry	143
Pike	140
Pork chuck	140
Veal, chop, cutlet with bone	140
Veal, fillet	140
Veal, shoulder	140
Fish, Haddock	139
Duck, average	138
Venison haunch (leg)	138
Pig's tongue	136
Scallop	136
Beef, muscles only	133
Rabbit meat, average with bone	132
Fish, Sole	131
Ham, cooked	131
Bean, seed, white, dry	128
Lentil, seed, dry	127
Pork belly, raw, smoked dried	127
Beef, chuck	120

Beef, fore rib, entrecote	120
Pork hip bone (hind leg)	120
Lobster	118
Chicken (chicken for roasting), average	115
Mussel	112
Sausage "Jagdwurst"	112
Beef, fillet	110
Beef, roast beef, sirloin	110
Beef, shoulder	110
Chicken, leg with skin, without bone	110
Fish, Pike-perch	110
Fish, Cod	109
Peas, chick (garbanzo), seed, dry	109
Grape, dried, raisin, sultana	107
Linseed	105
Rabbit/Hare (average)	105
Venison back	105
Sausage, salami, German	104
Sausages, frying, from pork	101
Pork belly	100

LOW PURITINE CONTENT 'Green' Foods	Total purines mg uric acid / 100 mg food (typical values)
Barley without husk, wholegrain	96
Sausage, "Mortadella"	96
Pea, seed, dry	95
Oats, without husk, wholegrain	94
Plaice	93
Calf's brain	92
Mushroom, flat, edible Boletus, cep	92
Sausages, frying, from veal	91
Oyster	90
Sausage, frankfurter	89
Sausage, "Bierschincken"	85
Pea, pod and seed, green	84
Pig's brain	83
Broccoli	81
Bean sprouts, Soya	80
Nuts, peanut	79
Artichoke	78
Fish, eel (smoked)	78
Sausage, "Fleischwurst"	78
Sausage, Vienna	78
Leek	74
Sausages, German (Mettwurst)	74
Apricot	73
Sausage, "Munich Weisswurst"	73
Grass, Viper's (black salsify)	71
Meat, luncheon	70
Brussel sprouts	69
Tofu	68

Chives	67
Fig, dried	64
Plum, dried	64
Millet, shucked corn	62
Sesame (gingelly) seed, Oriental, dry	62
Fish, Crayfish	60
Crispbread	60
Mushroom	58
Banana	57
Beef, corned (German)	57
Parsley, leaf	57
Spinach	57
Peppers, green	55
Pudding, black	55
Corn, sweet	52
Cauliflower	51
Rye, wholegrain	51
Wheat, wholegrain	51
Oyster, mushroom	50
Kale	48
Beans, French, dried	45
Pumpkin	44
Pasta made with egg (noodles, macaroni, spaghetti)	40
Lettuce, Lamb's	38
Almond, sweet	37
Beans, French (string beans, haricot)	37
Cabbage, savoy	37
Nuts, hazelnut (cobnut)	37
Date, dried	35
Elderberry, black	33
Melon, Cantelope	33

Cabbage, red	32
Cheese, Limburger, 20% fat content in dry matter	32
Celeriac	30
Quince	30
Bamboo shoots	29
Mushrooms, canned, solid and liquid	29
Olive, green, marinated	29
Cress	28
Grape	27
Kohlrabi	25
Nuts, Walnut	25
Plum	24
Squash, summer	24
Asparagus	23
Nuts, Brazil	23
Bilberry, blueberry	22
Cabbage, white	22
Aubergine	21
Peach	21
Rolls, bread	21
Strawberry	21
Avocado	19
Beetroot	19
Kiwi fruit (Chinese gooseberry, strawberry peach)	19
Orange	19
Pineapple	19
Potato, cooked with skin	18
Raspberry	18
Carrot	17
Cherry, Morello	17

Currant, red	17
Endive	17
Mushrooms, Chanterelle	17
Mushrooms, Chanterelles, canned, solids & liquid	17
Gooseberry	16
Potato	16
Sauerkraut	16
Radish	15
Apple	14
Beer, real, light	14
Bread, wheat (flour) or (white bread)	14
Fennel leaves	14
Beer, Pilsner lager beer, regular beer, German	13
Lettuce	13
Onion	13
Radishes	13
Chicory	12
Pear	12
Rhubarb	12
Tomato	11
Cheese, cottage	9.4
Beer, alcohol free	8.1
Yogurt, min. 3.5% fat content	8.1
Cucumber	7.3
Cheese, Brie	7.1
Cheese, edam	7.1
Cherry, sweet	7.1
Cheese, Cheddar/Cheshire cheese	6

Chapter 21

Good girls don't get gout:
the facts about gout in women...

FACT: one in five women over 60 suffer from gout.

The condition especially affects postmenopausal women.

Often the condition is misdiagnosed as osteoarthritis ('wear and tear' arthritis) because the possibility of gout in a woman is overlooked.

Until the appearance of the characteristic swelling of a joint, typically in the foot, accompanied by severe burning or stabbing pain occurs, the correct diagnosis may be missed.

Often the joint is not the typical one found in men – the big toe – but the ankle or a finger.

Women who consume foods high in purines, such as beef and seafood, or women with certain medical conditions, such as high blood pressure, and those who are taking thiazide diuretics (water pills) are especially prone to gout.

During the menopause, which on average occurs at age 52, a woman's body starts to produce dramatically less oestrogen.

Because oestrogen helps the kidneys to excrete uric acid, the lack of oestrogen results in increasing levels of blood uric acid which in turn leads to the formation of painful gout crystals in joints.

By the age of 60, the prevalence of gout in women is the same as in men, and by age 80, gout is more common in women than in men.

If you are a woman and a gout sufferer, then the same dietary advice as is described elsewhere in this book is important.

But that's not all.

Some women whose bodies produce too much uric acid may need medication in the form of allopurinol to reduce the formation of uric acid.

Other women's bodies don't excrete uric acid fast enough, and these women may benefit from a medication such as probenecid.

"I used to associate gout
with the ankles of a
degenerate great-grandfather;
I didn't realise it could also afflict
the wrists of the virtuous.
Now I know better."

Dervla Murphy, Irish travel writer

Part 4

Additional Resources Guide
(to help you overcome your gout pain)

UK Gout Society

http://www.ukgoutsociety.org/

The UK Gout Society is a registered charity and was established in 2002 to provide basic information to people living with gout, their families, friends and carers - and increase public awareness about this painful, potentially disabling, but very treatable, disorder.

Its trustee board comprises experienced rheumatologists and health professionals working in the field of gout.

The UK Gout Society is a member of ARMA (Arthritis and Musculoskeletal Alliance.

ARMA (Arthritis and Musculoskeletal Alliance)

http://arma.uk.net/

ARMA is the umbrella body providing a collective voice for the arthritis and musculoskeletal community in the UK.

Together, ARMA and its member organisations work to improve quality of life for around 10 million people in the UK with these conditions.

ARMA aims to foster co-operation between charities and professional organisations, working to enhance understanding and mutual support between individuals and organisational bodies.

Apps:

iGoutapp (for iOS)

by The University of Iowa (ITS)

This app is intended as a general reference for both health professionals and patients about gout and its management.

In addition to factual information, the app includes clinical, radiological and microscopic images as well as interactive case discussion and self-assessment questions.

Medications of choice are listed and are linked to PDR.

Gout Channel (for iOS)

By FBCommunication

Gout Channel optimises the best in digital technology to deliver dynamic and engaging professional and educational resources to your handheld device.

Thanks to an easy-to-navigate and intuitive interface, patients and healthcare professionals will be able to access dedicated content about Gout via iPad, iPhone or iPod touch – anytime, anywhere.

App Contents:

Patients:

- What is Gout?
- Why do I have Gout?
- What can I do about Gout?

Healthcare professionals:

- Gout treatments
- Videos
- Articles

Dynamic content:

Access a range of frequently updated content and resources via your handheld device. Download the App now and receive automatic notification of updates

Engaging multimedia:

Listen to the experts, watch videos, download images. New interactive features coming soon

Share resources:

Export content for personal use, or share information with colleagues and patients at the touch of a button

"No anatomist ever discovered a system of organization, calculated to produce pain and disease; or, in explaining the parts of the human body, ever said, this is to irritate; this is to inflame; this duct is to convey the gravel to the kidneys; this gland to secrete the humour which forms the gout: if by chance he come at a part of which he knows not the use, the most he can say is, that it is useless; no one ever suspects that it is put there to incommode, to annoy, or torment."

William Paley,
The Principles of Moral and Political Philosophy
(1785), Vol. 1, 79.

Conclusion – Final Words From Nick Wrathall

You've come to the end of your journey through our book *Goutbusters*.

But in effect, it's only the beginning...

What Dr Spira and I have given you in *Goutbusters* is a comprehensive guide to the causes of gout, and the simple measures you can take to relieve your gout pain.

As Dr Spira has outlined in *Goutbusters*, there is as yet no cure for gout. But that doesn't mean you have to suffer from gout pain for the rest of your life.

I've certainly benefited from what I've read in this comprehensive book, and although my gout attacks still occur, they're much less frequent than they used to be.

As with anything in life, there are always new ways to overcome a challenging health condition and gout is no different.

But more than anything, I want to get across to you that however bad your gout pain is right now, and whatever havoc it's wreaking in your life, you do have the possibility to reduce and even get rid of painful gout attacks for good.

Think for a moment what you could gain from using it. The possibility of a life of reduced pain, increased flexibility in your joints, being able to climb stairs and bend over without fear of the agonising pain you and I know all too well, doing things you thought you'd never do again: gardening; walking; playing with your grandchildren...

It may be something different, but I can't stress this enough: your situation is not hopeless, and by following Dr Spira's advice here in *Goutbusters*, you give yourself the chance to regain control of your life and body. I know this from personal experience.

That's got to be worth fighting for, hasn't it?

With our very best wishes for your future happiness and success, and a pain-free life.

Yours sincerely,

Nick Wrathall

Nick Wrathall
Editor, *Goutbusters*

P.S. As a special 'thank you', and to help you on your journey to a life free of gout pain, you also receive a free bonus gift (available to you as a *Goutbusters* owner).

Full details to claim your free gift are on the next page...

Special Free Gift From The Authors Of *Goutbusters*

To help you get even more value from this book, please take advantage of the FREE extra resource waiting for you at:

www.drgout.com

- Automatic membership to **The Dr Gout Digest** FREE enewsletter service

The Dr Gout Digest is your weekly email newsletter service, written exclusively for gout sufferers and those who love them.

Sent to you every Friday, each issue of **The Dr Gout Digest** contains details of the latest tips, techniques and strategies to help you relieve your gout pain, and shows you the medical breakthroughs the top health professionals worldwide use to make your life that little bit easier – and more gout free.

When it comes to getting rid of gout pain, you'll get to see what works best, what to avoid, and how to enjoy maximum pain relief in minimum time. And (most important of all) how you can conquer your gout attacks, regain control of your life, health and happiness, and enjoy yourself in the process...

Here's How To Activate Your Free Membership Of
The Dr Gout Digest enewsletter

1. Please go to the website at: www.drgout.com

2. Simply complete your name, address and email details in the spaces provided on this web page.

3. Once we receive these, you'll receive a confirmation email in your inbox. Just following the simple instructions in this email and your membership of **The Dr Gout Digest** enewsletter will be activated automatically.

4. **EXTRA MYSTERY BONUS GIFT**: when you activate your membership, you'll also receive an extra bonus gift (worth £10.00) and only available to members of *The Dr Gout Digest* enewsletter. Full details of how to obtain this when you join...

That's all there is to it! Look forward to seeing you there...

Yours sincerely,

Nick Wrathall

Nick Wrathall
Editor, *Goutbusters*

**** STOP PRESS ****

Could this new breakthrough be the answer to gout sufferers' prayers? See for yourself...

AstraZeneca may have a gout blockbuster on its hands with lesinurad

"With the rates of gout on the rise throughout the world, AstraZeneca ($AZN) and its Phase III therapy lesinurad could be lined up for a lead role in a growing market, welcome news for the sluggish pharma giant and its thin late-stage pipeline.

"As Bloomberg points out, the disease is on the rise in the West, afflicting 8.3 million Americans by 2011 and increasing 64% in the U.K. from 1997 to 2012, and roughly 17.7 million patients are expected to come down with gout by 2021, according to a study.

"Meanwhile, current treatments are limited to the 50-year-old generic allopurinol and Takeda and Ipsen's ($IPN) febuxostat, a drug approved in 2009that doesn't work in every patient, the news service notes.

"That sets the stage for AstraZeneca and its promising lesinurad. The drug is a selective uric acid re-absorption inhibitor that blocks the URAT1 transporter, treating the painful condition by normalizing acid excretion and reducing serum levels.

"In top-line results from a Phase III study on gout patients who get no benefit from allopurinol and febuxostat, lesinurad alone significantly reduced serum levels of uric acid, AstraZeneca said."

Full article at: http://www.fiercebiotech.com/story/astrazeneca-may-have-gout-blockbuster-its-hands-lesinurad/2014-02-14

Part 5

References & Resources

In *Goutbusters*, you've seen how gout is caused, and the simple, practical methods you can use to know for sure whether you have gout, and if so, the best ways to treat and/or prevent it.

Now for the "science" part!

To make sure you have all the information you need to make the best decisions for you and your health, I've included a comprehensive list of scientific and medical references and resources, to back up everything you've read in parts 1 and 2 of *Goutbusters*.

Reading through some of the many references can seem a little daunting, but rest assured they're worth their weight in gold.

This is because they're written by doctors, surgeons and medical practitioners at the cutting edge of gout research. In other words, gout experts who work with gout sufferers on a daily basis, at the cutting edge of the very latest medical research on the condition.

Although some of them are very technical, they contain many research papers and review articles and provide you with informative and interesting ways to combat gout when you suffer an attack, straight from the "horse's mouth" (i.e. the doctors on the front line of the war against gout).

So for this reason, it's definitely worth your while spending a little time on them. Plus, as with many important things in life, the more informed you are about the condition, the better you are able to manage and control it.

On the next page, I'm going to include a quick guide reference table, so you can read specific reports based on their conclusions (which are written in easy to understand terms)

With this in mind – and in the spirit of this book – please read the reports with an open mind, and I'm sure you'll be very pleasantly surprised. One thing is certain: the benefits to your health – and absence of gout – could be enormous.

Please turn over the page...

References & Resources – Quick Guide Table

THE BOTTOM LINE: Gout is on the increase, and much of it is due to diet and lifestyle.

Choi HK, Curhan G. Gout: epidemiology and lifestyle choices. Curr Opin Rheumatol. 2005;17(3):341–345.

Abstract

PURPOSE OF REVIEW:
Recent scientific data serve to illuminate the links between dietary and other factors and the incidence of gout. This review summarises recent literature about the prevalence and incidence of gout as well as risk factors for gout.

RECENT FINDINGS:
Epidemiologic studies suggest that the overall disease burden of gout is substantial and growing. Gout seems to be relatively common not only in men but also in older women.

A recent large prospective study investigated several purported dietary factors for gout and confirmed some of the long-standing suspicions (red meats, seafood, beer, and liquor), exonerated others (total protein, wine, and purine-rich vegetables), and also identified potentially new protective factors (dairy products).

A study based on the Third National Health and Nutrition Examination Survey suggested that these factors affect serum uric acid levels parallel to the direction of risk of gout. In addition, adiposity (i.e. being fat), weight gain, hypertension, and diuretics were all found to be independent risk factors for incident gout, whereas weight loss was found to be protective.

SUMMARY:
The disease burden of gout remains substantial and may be increasing. Some of the recently confirmed lifestyle factors may explain the increasing incidence of gout. The public health implications of dietary and lifestyle recommendations should take into account other

associated health benefits and risks, because many of these factors have health effects beyond their influence on gout.

Nriagu JO. Saturnine gout among Roman aristocrats. Did lead poisoning contribute to the fall of the Empire? N Engl J Med. 1983;308(11):660–663.

Healey LA. Port wine and the gout. Arthritis Rheum. 1975;18(Suppl 6):659–662.

Steinbock RT. Lead ingestion in history. N Engl J Med. 1979;301(5):277.

Martinon F, Glimcher LH; Gout: new insights into an old disease. J Clin Invest. 2006 Aug;116(8):2073-5.

Nuki G., Simkin P.A. A concise history of gout and hyperuricemia and their treatment. Arthritis Res. Ther. 2006;8(Suppl. 1):S1.

Dalbeth N., Haskard D.O. Mechanisms of inflammation in gout. Rheumatology (Oxford). 2005;44:1090–1096.

Faires J.S., McCarty D.J. Acute arthritis in man and dog after intrasynovial infection of sodium urate crystals. Lancet. 1962;280:682–685.

Richette P, Bardin T (January 2010). "Gout". Lancet 375 (9711): 318–28. doi:10.1016/S0140-6736(09)60883-7.

Stephen E. Malawista, Anne Chevance de Boisfleury, Paul H. Naccache. Inflammatory Gout: Observations over a Half-Century. FASEB J. 2011 December; 25(12): 4073–4078. doi: 10.1096/fj.11-1201ufm.

Pillinger, MH; Rosenthal P, Abeles AM (2007). "Hyperuricemia and gout: new insights into pathogenesis and treatment". Bulletin of the NYU Hospital for Joint Diseases 65 (3): 215–221. PMID 17922673.

"The Disease Of Kings - Forbes.com". Forbes.

Roddy E. Revisiting the pathogenesis of podagra: why does gout target the foot? J Foot Ankle Res2011;4:13.

Roddy E, Doherty M. Epidemiology of gout. Arthritis Res Ther2010;12:223.

FICTION: Only overweight wealthy people get gout.

FACT: People of all shapes and sizes get gout, although the risk increases if you're overweight or obese.

THE BOTTOM LINE: 10 scientifically validated diagnostic tests for gout.

Zhang W, Doherty M, Pascual E, Bardin T, Barskova V, Conaghan P, et al; EULAR Standing Committee for International Clinical Studies Including Therapeutics. EULAR evidence based recommendations for gout. Part I: diagnosis. Report of a task force of the Standing Committee for International Clinical Studies Including Therapeutics (ESCISIT). Ann Rheum Dis2006;65:1301-11.

Abstract

OBJECTIVE:
To develop evidence based recommendations for the diagnosis of gout.

METHODS:
The multidisciplinary guideline development group comprised 19 rheumatologists and one evidence based medicine expert, representing 13 European countries. Ten key propositions regarding diagnosis were generated using a Delphi consensus approach. Research evidence was searched systematically for each proposition.

Wherever possible the sensitivity, specificity, likelihood ratio (LR), and incremental cost-effectiveness ratio were calculated for diagnostic tests.

Relative risk and odds ratios were estimated for risk factors and co-morbidities associated with gout.

The quality of evidence was categorised according to the evidence hierarchy. The strength of recommendation (SOR) was assessed using the EULAR visual analogue and ordinal scales.

RESULTS:

10 key propositions were generated though three Delphi rounds including diagnostic topics in clinical manifestations, urate crystal identification, biochemical tests, radiographs, and risk factors/co-morbidities.

Urate crystal identification varies according to symptoms and observer skill but is very likely to be positive in symptomatic gout (LR = 567 (95% confidence interval (CI), 35.5 to 9053)).

Classic podagra and presence of tophi have the highest clinical diagnostic value for gout (LR = 30.64 (95% CI, 20.51 to 45.77), and LR = 39.95 (21.06 to 75.79), respectively).

Hyperuricaemia (a very high level of uric acid in the blood) is a major risk factor for gout and may be a useful diagnostic marker when defined by the normal range of the local population (LR = 9.74 (7.45 to 12.72)), although some gouty patients may have normal serum uric acid concentrations at the time of investigation.

Radiographs have little role in diagnosis, though in late or severe gout radiographic changes of asymmetrical swelling (LR = 4.13 (2.97 to 5.74)) and subcortical cysts without erosion (LR = 6.39 (3.00 to 13.57)) may be useful to differentiate chronic gout from other joint conditions.

In addition, risk factors (sex, diuretics, purine-rich foods, alcohol, lead) and co-morbidities (cardiovascular diseases, hypertension, diabetes, obesity, and chronic renal failure) are associated with gout. SOR for each proposition varied according to both the research evidence and expert opinion.

CONCLUSIONS:

10 key recommendations for diagnosis of gout were developed using a combination of research based evidence and expert consensus. The evidence for diagnostic tests, risk factors, and co-morbidities was evaluated and the strength of recommendation was provided.

THE BOTTOM LINE: 12 key recommendations for the management of gout.

Zhang W, Doherty M, Pascual E, Bardin T, Barskova V, Conaghan P, et al; EULAR Standing Committee for International Clinical Studies Including Therapeutics. EULAR evidence based recommendations for gout. Part II: management. Report of a task force of the Standing Committee for International Clinical Studies Including Therapeutics (ESCISIT). Ann Rheum Dis2006;65:1312-24.

Abstract

OBJECTIVE:
To develop evidence based recommendations for the management of gout.

METHODS:
The multidisciplinary guideline development group comprised 19 rheumatologists and one evidence based medicine expert representing 13 European countries. Key propositions on management were generated using a Delphi consensus approach. Research evidence was searched systematically for each proposition. Where possible, effect size (ES), number needed to treat, relative risk, odds ratio, and incremental cost-effectiveness ratio were calculated. The quality of evidence was categorised according to the level of evidence. The strength of recommendation (SOR) was assessed using the EULAR visual analogue and ordinal scales.

RESULTS:
12 key propositions were generated after three Delphi rounds.

Propositions included both non-pharmacological and pharmacological treatments and addressed symptomatic control of acute gout, urate lowering therapy (ULT), and prophylaxis of acute attacks.

The importance of patient education, modification of adverse lifestyle (weight loss if obese; reduced alcohol consumption; low animal purine diet) and treatment of associated comorbidity and risk factors were emphasised.

Recommended drugs for acute attacks were oral non-steroidal anti-inflammatory drugs (NSAIDs), oral colchicine (ES = 0.87 (95% confidence interval, 0.25 to 1.50)), or joint aspiration and injection of corticosteroid.

ULT is indicated in patients with recurrent acute attacks, arthropathy, tophi, or radiographic changes of gout.

Allopurinol was confirmed as effective long term ULT (ES = 1.39 (0.78 to 2.01)). If allopurinol toxicity occurs, options include other xanthine oxidase inhibitors, allopurinol desensitisation, or a uricosuric.

The uricosuric benzbromarone is more effective than allopurinol (ES = 1.50 (0.76 to 2.24)) and can be used in patients with mild to moderate renal insufficiency but may be hepatotoxic.

When gout is associated with the use of diuretics, the diuretic should be stopped if possible. For prophylaxis the best treatment to give against acute attacks, either colchicine 0.5-1 mg daily or an NSAID (with gastroprotection if indicated) are recommended.

CONCLUSIONS:
12 key recommendations for management of gout were developed, using a combination of research based evidence and expert consensus. The evidence was evaluated and the SOR provided for each proposition.

THE BOTTOM LINE: Contrary to other research, gout doesn't seem to have become more common in recent years.

Edwards NL. The role of hyperuricemia and gout in kidney and cardiovascular disease. Cleveland Clin J Med2008;75:S13-16.

Mikuls TR, Farrar JT, Bilker WB, Fernandes S, Schumacher HR Jr, Saag KG. Gout epidemiology: results from the UK General Practice Research Database, 1990–1999. Ann Rheum Dis2005;64:267-72.

Abstract

OBJECTIVE:
To examine the epidemiology (the science and study of the patterns, causes, and effects of health and disease) of gout and gout treatment in the United Kingdom using a large national practice based population.

METHODS:
Data from the UK General Practice Research Database from 1990 to 1999 were examined. Physician diagnoses and drug codes were used, and trends in gout incidence and treatment examined. Additionally, disease prevalence for the year 1999 was assessed.

To examine the association of gout with comorbid disease, the prevalence of select health conditions and drug use was compared with the corresponding prevalences seen in osteoarthritis, adjusting for both age and sex.

RESULTS:
From 1 January 1990 to 31 December 1999 overall gout incidence remained relatively stable, ranging from a low of 11.9 cases (95% confidence interval (CI) 11.5 to 12.3) in 1991 to a high of 18.0 cases (95% CI 17.6 to 18.4) per 10 000 patient-years in 1994.

Gout prevalence in 1999 was 1.4% with rates approaching 7% in men over the age of 65.

Drugs used for the treatment of gout remained constant in prevalent cases with the exception of a significant decline in non-steroidal anti-inflammatory drug use over the 10 year follow up.

Compared with patients with osteoarthritis, patients with gout were significantly more likely to have cardiovascular disease, hypertension, diabetes, and chronic renal failure, and were more likely to have used diuretics or ciclosporin, or both.

CONCLUSION: Although gout is common in the UK, particularly among older men, the incidence of the disease seems to have remained stable during the 1990s.

FICTION: Women don't get gout – only men.

FACT: Both men and women can suffer from gout, although men are more likely to be afflicted. Gout is 10 times more common in men than in women, until women reach menopause. After the age of 60, new gout cases in men and women tend to be about the same.

THE BOTTOM LINE: In treating gout it is important to manage correctly co-existing conditions such as diabetes and heart failure.

Zhu Y, Pandya BJ, Choi HK. Comorbidities of gout and hyperuricemia in the US general population: NHANES 2007-2008. Am J Med2012;125:679-687.e1.

Abstract

PURPOSE:
The objective of this study was to estimate the latest prevalence of major comorbidities (the presence of one or more disorders in addition to a primary disease or disorder, or the effect of such additional disorders or diseases) associated with gout and hyperuricemia in the US based on a recent, nationally representative sample of US men and women.

METHODS:
Using data from 5,707 participants aged 20 years and older in the National Health and Nutrition Examination Survey 2007-2008, we calculated the national prevalence and population estimates of major comorbidities according to gout status and various hyperuricemia levels, compared with those without these conditions.

Case definitions of gout and comorbidities were based on an affirmative answer to a question that asked whether a physician or a health professional had diagnosed the corresponding condition.

RESULTS:
Among these individuals with gout,

- 74% (6.1 million) had hypertension

- 71% (5.5 million) had chronic kidney disease stage ≥2

- 53% (4.3 million) were obese

- 26% (2.1 million) had diabetes

- 24% (2.0 million) had nephrolithiasis (a condition in which hard masses (kidney stones) form within the urinary tract)

- 14% (1.2 million) had myocardial infarction

- 11% (0.9 million) had heart failure

- 10% (0.9 million) had suffered a stroke

These proportions were substantially higher than those among individuals without gout (all P-values <.67). With increasing levels of hyperuricemia, there were graded increases in the prevalences of these comorbidities. In the top category (serum urate ≥10 mg/dL), 86% of subjects had chronic kidney disease stage ≥2, 66% had hypertension, 65% were obese, 33% had heart failure, 33% had diabetes, 23% had myocardial infarction, and 12% had stroke.

These prevalences were 3-33 times higher than those in the lowest serum urate category (<4 mg/dL). Sex-specific odds ratios tended to be larger among women than men, and the overall comorbidity prevalence was highest among individuals with both gout and hyperuricemia.

CONCLUSIONS:
These findings from the latest nationally representative data highlight remarkable prevalences and population estimates of comorbidities of gout and hyperuricemia in the US.

Appropriate preventive and management measures of these comorbidities should be implemented in gout management, with a preference to strategies that can improve gout and comorbidities together.

THE BOTTOM LINE: There is a high incidence of metabolic syndrome (the combination of diabetes, high blood pressure and obesity) in patients with gout, and it is important to recognise this fact in the management of gout.

Choi HK, Ford ES, Li C, Curhan G. Prevalence of the metabolic syndrome in patients with gout: the third national health and nutrition examination survey. Arthritis Rheum2007;57:109-15.

Abstract

OBJECTIVE:
To determine the prevalence of metabolic syndrome (the medical term for a combination of diabetes, high blood pressure and obesity) among patients with gout and to examine the association between the two conditions in a nationally representative sample of US adults.

METHODS:
Using data from 8,807 participants age >or=20 years in the Third National Health and Nutrition Examination Survey (1988-1994), we determined the prevalence of metabolic syndrome among individuals with gout and quantified the magnitude of association between the two conditions.

We used both the revised and original National Cholesterol Education Program Adult Treatment Panel III (NCEP/ATP III) criteria to define metabolic syndrome.

RESULTS:
The prevalence (95% confidence interval [95% CI]) of metabolic syndrome according to revised NCEP/ATP III criteria was 62.8% (51.9-73.6) among individuals with gout and 25.4% (23.5-27.3) among individuals without gout. Using 2002 census data, approximately 3.5 million US adults with a history of gout have metabolic syndrome.

The unadjusted and age- and sex-adjusted odds ratios (95% CI) of metabolic syndrome for individuals with gout were 4.96 (3.17-

7.75) and 3.05 (2.01-4.61), respectively. With the original NCEP/ATP criteria, the corresponding prevalences were slightly lower, whereas the corresponding odds ratios were slightly higher.

The stratified prevalences of metabolic syndrome by major associated factors of gout (i.e. body mass index, hypertension, and diabetes) remained substantially and significantly higher among those with gout than those without gout (all P values <0.05).

CONCLUSION:
These findings indicate that the prevalence of metabolic syndrome is remarkably high among individuals with gout. Given the serious complications associated with metabolic syndrome, this frequent comorbidity should be recognised and taken into account in long-term treatment and overall health of individuals with gout.

FICTION: Gout pain always attacks the big toe.

FACT: Although gout often first attacks the big toe joints, it's not the only 'first port of call', and can also strike in the ankles, feet and joints of the hands. The first attacks often attack one or two joints, but if it isn't treated, then gout can spread to multiple joints and cause permanent damage.

FICTION: Don't eat any meat or drink any alcohol and you'll never suffer gout attacks.

FACT: Alcoholic drinks — especially beer and spirits — and so-called 'organ meats' (which include liver and fish such as anchovies and sardines) are, as you already know, purines, which create uric acid. But although avoiding certain types of meat, fish and alcohol may reduce attacks, it won't stop them completely, as others factors such as heredity and stress are known causes of gout.

THE BOTTOM LINE: Alcohol, especially beer, is strongly associated with an increased risk of gout, although moderate wine consumption does not increase the risk.

PMID: 17266099 [PubMed - indexed for MEDLINE]

Choi HK, Atkinson K, Karlson EW, Willett W, Curhan G. Alcohol intake and risk of incident gout in men: a prospective study. Lancet 2004;363:1277-81.

Abstract

BACKGROUND:
The association between alcohol consumption and risk of gout has been suspected since ancient times, but has not been prospectively confirmed. Additionally, potential differences in risk of gout posed by different alcoholic beverages have not been assessed.

METHODS:
Over 12 years (1986-98) we used biennial questionnaires to investigate the relation between alcohol consumption and risk of incident gout in 47,150 male participants with no history of gout at baseline. We used a supplementary questionnaire to ascertain whether reported cases of gout met the American College of Rheumatology survey gout criteria.

FINDINGS:
We documented 730 confirmed incident cases of gout. Compared with men who did not drink alcohol, the multivariate relative risk (RR) of gout was 1.32 (95% CI 0.99-1.75) for alcohol consumption 10.0-14.9 g/day, 1.49 (1.14-1.94) for 15.0-29.9 g/day, 1.96 (1.48-2.60) for 30.0-49.9 g/day, and 2.53 (1.73-3.70) for > or =50 g/day (p for trend <0.0001).

Beer consumption showed the strongest independent association with the risk of gout (multivariate RR per 12-oz serving per day 1.49; 95% CI 1.32-1.70).

Consumption of spirits was also significantly associated with gout (multivariate RR per drink or shot per day 1.15; 95% CI 1.04-1.28); however, wine consumption was not (multivariate RR per 4-oz serving per day 1.04; 95% CI 0.88-1.22).

INTERPRETATION:

Alcohol intake is strongly associated with an increased risk of gout. This risk varies substantially according to type of alcoholic beverage: beer confers a larger risk than spirits, whereas moderate wine drinking does not increase the risk.

FICTION: Gout is very painful, but not fatal.

FACT: Whilst it's certainly true that gout can't kill you immediately, it can cause serious health problems that may eventually kill you. For example, it can increase your susceptibility to heart attacks or strokes. If gout is untreated, tophi can develop, which in turn can become infected and prove to be life-threatening.

THE BOTTOM LINE: Eating lots of meat and seafood is associated with an increased risk of gout, whereas dairy products are associated with a decreased risk.

Choi HK, Atkinson K, Karlson EW, Willett W, Curhan G. Purine-rich foods, dairy and protein intake, and the risk of gout in men. N Engl J Med 2004;350:1093-103.

Abstract

BACKGROUND:

Various purine-rich foods and high protein intake have long been thought to be risk factors for gout. Similarly, the possibility that the consumption of dairy products has a role in protecting against gout has been raised by metabolic studies. We prospectively investigated the association of these dietary factors with new cases of gout.

METHODS:

Over a 12-year period, we prospectively examined the relationship between purported dietary risk factors and new cases of gout among 47,150 men who had no history of gout at baseline.

We used a supplementary questionnaire to ascertain whether participants met the American College of Rheumatology survey criteria for gout. Diet was assessed every four years by means of a food-frequency questionnaire.

RESULTS:

During the 12 years of the study, we documented 730 confirmed new cases of gout. The multivariate relative risk of gout among men in the highest quintile of meat intake, as compared with those in the lowest quintile, was 1.41 (i.e. those who were in the top 20% of meat consumption suffered from a 41% higher incidence of gout than those in the lowest 20% of meat conmsumption) (95 percent confidence interval, 1.07 to 1.86; P for trend = 0.02), and the corresponding relative risk associated with seafood intake was 1.51 (95 percent confidence interval, 1.17 to 1.95; P for trend = 0.02).

In contrast, the incidence of gout decreased with increasing intake of dairy products; the multivariate relative risk among men in the highest quintile, as compared with those in the lowest quintile, was 0.56 (95 percent confidence interval, 0.42 to 0.74; P for trend <0.001).

The level of consumption of purine-rich vegetables and the total protein intake were not associated with an increased risk of gout.

CONCLUSIONS:
Higher levels of meat and seafood consumption are associated with an increased risk of gout, whereas a higher level of consumption of dairy products is associated with a decreased risk. Moderate intake of purine-rich vegetables or protein is not associated with an increased risk of gout.

FICTION: There are no effective medicines for preventing gout from occurring.

FACT: As you have seen, this is not true. As already discussed, you have Naproxen and Colchicine (Colcrys) for acute gout flare-ups. Then there are the drugs which regulate the levels of uric acid in your blood, such as allopurinol and febuxostat.

THE BOTTOM LINE: Sugar sweetened soft drinks, fructose, fructose rich fruits and fruit juices are associated with an increased risk of gout in men, whereas diet soft drinks are not associated with an increased risk.

Choi HK, Curhan G. Soft drinks, fructose consumption, and the risk of gout in men: prospective cohort study. BMJ2008;336:309-12.

Abstract

OBJECTIVE:
To examine the relation between intake of sugar sweetened soft drinks and fructose and the risk of incident gout in men.

DESIGN:
Prospective cohort (medical study) over 12 years.

SETTING:
Health professionals follow-up study.

PARTICIPANTS:
46,393 men with no history of gout at baseline who provided information on intake of soft drinks and fructose through validated food-frequency questionnaires.

MAIN OUTCOME MEASURE:
Incident cases of gout meeting the American College of Rheumatology survey criteria for gout.

RESULTS:
During the 12 years of follow-up, 755 confirmed incident cases of gout were reported.

Increasing intake of sugar sweetened soft drinks was associated with an increasing risk of gout. Compared with consumption of less than one serving of sugar sweetened soft drinks a month, the multivariate relative risk of gout for 5-6 servings a week was 1.29 (95% confidence interval 1.00 to 1.68), for one serving a day was 1.45 (1.02 to 2.08), and for two or more servings a day was 1.85 (1.08 to 3.16; P for trend=0.002).

Diet soft drinks were not associated with risk of gout (P for trend=0.99). The multivariate relative risk of gout according to increasing fifths of fructose intake were 1.00, 1.29, 1.41, 1.84, and 2.02 (1.49 to 2.75; P for trend <0.001).

Other major contributors to fructose intake such as total fruit juice or fructose rich fruits (apples and oranges) were also associated with a higher risk of gout (P values for trend <0.05).

CONCLUSIONS:

Prospective data suggest that consumption of sugar sweetened soft drinks and fructose is strongly associated with an increased risk of gout in men. Furthermore, fructose rich fruits and fruit juices may also increase the risk. Diet soft drinks were not associated with the risk of gout.

FICTION: Making changes to your lifestyle make no difference to relieving gout pain.

FACT: Not true. Eating the right foods, eliminating or cutting down on the consumption of high-purine foods (and replacing them with vegetable proteins such as beans and peas), drinking less alcohol, taking exercise and losing weight will all have a positive effect on reducing both the frequency and severity of your gout attacks.

THE BOTTOM LINE: Coffee seems to have a protective effect for gout.

Choi HK, Willett W, Curhan G. Coffee consumption and risk of incident gout in men: a prospective study. Arthritis Rheum2007;56:2049-55.

Abstract

OBJECTIVE:
Coffee is one of the most widely consumed beverages in the world and may affect the risk of gout via various mechanisms. We prospectively evaluated the relationship between coffee intake and the risk of incident gout in a large cohort of men.

METHODS:
Over a 12-year period, we studied 45,869 men with no history of gout at baseline. Intake of coffee, decaffeinated coffee, tea, and total caffeine was assessed every four years through validated questionnaires. We used a supplementary questionnaire to ascertain whether participants met the American College of Rheumatology survey criteria for gout.

RESULTS:
We documented 757 confirmed incident cases of gout. Increasing coffee intake was inversely associated with the risk of gout (i.e. the more coffee you drink, the lower the risk of gout).

The multivariate relative risks (RRs) for incident gout according to coffee consumption categories (0, <1, 1-3, 4-5, and > or = 6 cups per day) were 1.00, 0.97, 0.92, 0.60 (95% confidence interval [95% CI] 0.41-0.87), and 0.41 (95% CI 0.19-0.88), respectively (P for trend = 0.009).

For decaffeinated coffee, the multivariate RRs according to consumption categories (0, <1, 1-3, and > or = 4 cups per day) were 1.00, 0.83, 0.67 (95% CI 0.54-0.82), and 0.73 (95% CI 0.46-1.17), respectively (P for trend = 0.002). Total caffeine from all sources and tea intake were not associated with the risk of gout.

CONCLUSION:

These prospective data suggest that long-term coffee consumption is associated with a lower risk of incident gout.

FICTION: If you ignore gout pain, sooner or later it will go away.

FACT: Even though gout attacks stop eventually, they're more likely to re-occur with greater frequency if you do nothing to stop them. So it's important to put together a long-term strategy, based on lifestyle, diet, exercise and the appropriate medication to cut the number of gout attacks.

THE BOTTOM LINE: Although certain diuretics are associated with a higher risk of acute gout, there is no good evidence for stopping these drugs in patients who develop gout.

Merriman TR, Dalbeth N. The genetic basis of hyperuricaemia and gout. Joint Bone Spine2011;78:35-40.

Hueskes BA, Roovers EA, Mantel-Teeuwisse AK, Janssens HJ, van de Lisdonk EH, Janssen M. Use of diuretics and the risk of gouty arthritis: a systematic review. Semin Arthritis Rheum2012;41:879-89.

Abstract

OBJECTIVE:
To systematically review the literature investigating the relationship between use of diuretics and the risk of gouty arthritis.

METHODS:
PubMed (1950-October 2009), Embase (1974-October 2009), and the Cochrane Library (up to October 2009) were searched using keywords and MeSH terms diuretics, adverse effects, and gout. For this review, the technique of "best evidence synthesis" was used.

Studies reporting frequency, absolute or relative risks, odds ratio, or rate ratio of gouty arthritis in diuretic users compared with non-users were selected and evaluated. Studies had to be published in English. Checklists from the Dutch Cochrane Centre were used to assess the quality of randomised controlled trials (RCTs), cohort, and case-control studies.

RESULTS:
Two RCTs, six cohort studies, and five case-control studies met the inclusion criteria. The overall quality of the studies was moderate. In a RCT the rate ratio of gout for use of bendrofluazide vs placebo was 11.8 (95% CI 5.2-27.0). The other RCT found a rate ratio of 6.3 (95% CI 0.8-51) for use of hydrochlorothiazide plus triamterene vs placebo. Three cohort studies and four case-control studies found higher risks of gouty arthritis in users compared with non-users of diuretics.

CONCLUSIONS:

There is a trend toward a higher risk for acute gouty arthritis attacks in patients on loop and thiazide diuretics, but the magnitude and independence is not consistent. Therefore, stopping these useful drugs in patients who develop gouty arthritis is not supported by the results of this review.

FICTION: Gout is only a mild form of arthritis.

FACT: Wrong. Gout has been described as the nearest a man will come to experiencing the pain of childbirth! And as already discussed, the long-term consequences of gout can prove to be fatal.

THE BOTTOM LINE: Many patients with gout fail to follow dietary guidelines.

Shulten P, Thomas J, Miller M, Smith M, Ahern M. The role of diet in the management of gout: a comparison of knowledge and attitudes to current evidence.

J Hum Nutr Diet. 2009 Feb;22(1):3-11. doi: 10.1111/j.1365-277X.2008.00928.x.

Abstract

BACKGROUND:
Evidence supports dietary modifications in the management of gout. Despite this, the degree of implementation of this evidence by nutrition professionals and rheumatologists and those affected by gout is unknown.

The present study aimed to compare usual dietary practices of patients with gout to evidence for dietary management of gout and to investigate whether the knowledge and attitudes of nutrition professionals and rheumatologists reflects current evidence.

METHODS:
A food-frequency questionnaire was used to determine usual dietary intake of patients with gout, a separate questionnaire examined gout-related dietary modifications (n = 29). Online questionnaires to examine attitudes towards dietary management of gout were completed by nutrition professionals and rheumatologists.

RESULTS:
Proportions of participants whose reported intakes were inconsistent with current evidence for the dietary management of gout were: alcohol, n = 14 (48%); beer, n = 18 (62%); seafood, n = 29 (100%); meat, n = 7 (24%); beef/pork/lamb, n = 24 (83%); dairy products, n = 12 (41%); vitamin C supplementation, n = 29 (100%).

Of the 61 rheumatologists and 231 nutrition professionals who completed the online survey, the majority considered that weight loss and decreased alcohol intake were important or very important outcomes. Proportions were lower for decreased purine intake. Thirty-four (56%) rheumatologists do not refer patients with gout to dietetic services and, of those who do, the majority refer less than half.

CONCLUSIONS:
Overall, patients with gout in the present study were not implementing evidence for dietary management of their condition and complex dietary issues were evident.

Roddy E, Mallen CD, Hider SL, Jordan KP. Prescription and comorbidity screening following consultation for acute gout in primary care. Rheumatol (Oxford)2010;49:105-11.

Brauer GW, Prior IA. A prospective study of gout in New Zealand Maoris. Ann Rheum Dis1978;37:466-72. Abstract/FREE Full Text

Goldthwait JC, Butler CF, Stillman JS. The diagnosis of gout; significance of an elevated serum uric acid value. N Engl J Med1958;259:1095-9. MedlineWeb of Science

Urano W, Yamanaka H, Tsutani H, Nakajima H, Matsuda Y, Taniguchi A, et al. The inflammatory process in the mechanism of decreased serum uric acid concentrations during acute gouty arthritis. J Rheumatol 2002;29:1950-3.

Chowalloor PV, Keen HI. A systematic review of ultrasonography in gout and asymptomatic hyperuricaemia. Ann Rheum Dis2013;72:638-45. Abstract/FREE Full Text

THE BOTTOM LINE: Gouty arthritis, caused by long-term high blood levels of uric acid, often occurs both inside and outside joints of patients who do not have symptoms of gout.

Pineda C, Amezcua-Guerra LM, Solano C, et al. Joint and tendon subclinical involvement suggestive of gouty arthritis in asymptomatic hyperuricemia: an ultrasound controlled study. Arthritis Res Ther2011;13:R4.

Abstract

INTRODUCTION:
In this study, we aimed to investigate ultrasonographic (US) changes suggestive of gouty arthritis in the hyaline cartilage, joints and tendons from asymptomatic individuals with hyperuricemia.

METHODS:
We conducted a cross-sectional, controlled study including US examinations of the knees and first metatarsal-phalangeal joints (first MTPJs), as well as of the tendons and enthesis of the lower limbs. Differences were estimated by χ^2 or unpaired t-tests as appropriate. Associations were calculated using the Spearman's correlation coefficient rank test.

RESULTS:
Fifty asymptomatic individuals with hyperuricemia and 52 normouricemic subjects were included. Hyperechoic enhancement of the superficial margin of the hyaline cartilage (double contour sign) was found in 25% of the first MTPJs from hyperuricemic individuals, in contrast to none in the control group (P < 0.0001).

Similar results were found on the femoral cartilage (17% versus 0; P < 0.0001). Patellar enthesopathy (12% versus 2.9%; P = 0.01) and tophi (6% versus 0; P = 0.01) as well as Achilles enthesopathy (15% versus 1.9%; P = 0.0007) were more frequent in hyperuricemic than in normouricemic individuals. Intra-articular tophi were found in eight hyperuricemic individuals but in none of the normouricemic subjects (P = 0.003).

CONCLUSIONS:

These data demonstrate that morphostructural changes suggestive of gouty arthritis induced by chronic hyperuricemia frequently occur in both intra- and extra-articular structures of clinically asymptomatic individuals.

FICTION: Only a few elderly, fat men suffer from gout.

FACT: Over two million UK and over eight million US citizens are known to suffer from gout. In fact, according to an article on page 138, Advances In Gerontology, Volume 3, No.2 2013 :

"Gout affects over 1% of the world's adult population and, furthermore, gout is the form of inflammatory arthritis most prevalent in men."

THE BOTTOM LINE: All drugs used to treat gout can have serious side effects. This is especially important in the elderly who are most at risk of gout.

De Miguel E, Puig JG, Castillo C, et al. Diagnosis of gout in patients with asymptomatic hyperuricaemia: a pilot ultrasound study. Ann Rheum Dis2012;71:157-8.

Sutaria S, Katbamna R, Underwood M. Effectiveness of interventions for the treatment of acute and prevention of recurrent gout - a systematic review. Rheumatol (Oxford)2006;45:1422-31.

Abstract

OBJECTIVE:
To determine the evidence for the effectiveness of treatments for acute gout and the prevention of recurrent gout.

METHOD:
Seven electronic databases were searched for randomised controlled trials of treatments for gout from their inception to the end of 2004. No language restrictions were applied. All randomised controlled trials of treatments routinely available for the treatment of gout were included. Trials of the prevention of recurrence were included only if patients who had had gout and had at least six months of follow-up were studied.

RESULTS:
We found 13 randomised controlled trials of treatment for acute gout, two of which were placebo controlled.

Colchicine was found to be effective in one study; however, the entire colchicine group developed toxicity.

The only robust conclusion from studies of non-steroidal anti-inflammatory drugs is that pain relief from indometacin and etoricoxib are equivalent. We found one randomised controlled trial, reported only as a conference abstract, of recurrent gout prevention.

CONCLUSION:

The shortage of robust data to inform the management of a common problem such as gout is surprising. All of the drugs used to treat gout can have serious side effects.

The incidence of gout is highest in the elderly population. It is in this group, who are at a high risk of serious adverse events, that we are using drugs of known toxicity. The balance of risks and benefits for the drug treatment of gout needs to be reassessed.

FICTION: Gout attacks come and go very quickly, and are over within 24 hours.

FACT: As a general rule, gout attacks last anything from one to seven days, but in extreme cases they can continue beyond the usual seven days and can result in serious damage to the joints.

THE BOTTOM LINE: A look at various ways of treating gout with prescribed medications.

Schumacher HR Jr, Boice JA, Daikh DI, Mukhopadhyay S, Malmstrom K, Ng J, et al. Randomised double blind trial of etoricoxib and indometacin in treatment of acute gouty arthritis. BMJ2002;324:1488-92. Abstract/ FREE Full Text

Rubin BR, Burton R, Navarra S, Antigua J, Londoño J, Pryhuber KG, et al. Efficacy and safety profile of treatment with etoricoxib 120 mg once daily compared with indomethacin 50 mg three times daily in acute gout: a randomized controlled trial. Arthritis Rheum2004;50:598-606. CrossRefMedlineWeb of Science

Man CY, Cheung IT, Cameron PA, Rainer TH. Comparison of oral prednisolone/paracetamol and oral indomethacin/paracetamol combination therapy in the treatment of acute goutlike arthritis: a double-blind, randomized, controlled trial. Ann Emerg Med2007;49:670-7. CrossRefMedlineWeb of Science

Janssens HJ, Janssen M, van de Lisdonk EH, van Riel PL, van Weel C. Use of oral prednisolone or naproxen for the treatment of gout arthritis: a double-blind, randomised equivalence trial. Lancet2008;371:1854-60. CrossRefMedlineWeb of Science

Khanna D, Khanna PP, Fitzgerald JD, Singh MK, Mae S, Neogi T et al. 2012 American College of Rheumatology guidelines for management of gout. Part 2: therapy and anti-inflammatory prophylaxis of acute gouty arthritis. Arthritis Care Res2012;64:1447-61.Web of Science.

- An acute gouty arthritis attack should be treated with pharmacologic therapy, initiated within 24 hours of onset.

- Established pharmacologic urate-lowering therapy should be continued, without interruption, during an acute attack of gout.

- Nonsteroidal anti-inflammatory drugs (NSAIDs), corticosteroids, or oral colchicine are appropriate first-line options for treatment of acute gout, and certain combinations can be employed for severe or refractory attacks.

- Pharmacologic anti-inflammatory prophylaxis is recommended for all gout patients when pharmacologic urate lowering is initiated, and should be continued if there is any clinical evidence of continuing gout disease activity and/or the serum urate target has not yet been achieved.

- Oral colchicine is an appropriate first-line gout attack prophylaxis therapy, including with appropriate dose adjustment in chronic kidney disease and for drug interactions, unless there is a lack of tolerance or medical contraindication.

- Low-dose NSAID therapy is an appropriate choice for first-line gout attack prophylaxis, unless there is a lack of tolerance or medical contraindication.

Ahern MJ, Reid C, Gordon TP, McCredie M, Brooks PM, Jones M. Does colchicine work? The results of the first controlled study in acute gout. Aust N Z J Med1987;17:301-4. CrossRefMedlineWeb of Science

Terkeltaub RA, Furst DE, Bennett K, Kook KA, Crockett RS, Davis MW. High versus low dosing of oral colchicine for early acute gout flare: twenty-four-hour outcome of the first multicenter, randomized, double-blind, placebo-controlled, parallel-group, dose-comparison colchicine study. Arthritis Rheum2010;62:1060-8. CrossRefMedline

THE BOTTOM LINE: Ice is a useful first aid treatment to reduce the pain of acute gout.

Schlesinger N, Detry MA, Holland BK, Baker DG, Beutler AM, Rull M, et al. Local ice therapy during bouts of acute gouty arthritis. J Rheumatol2002;29:331-4.

Abstract

OBJECTIVE:
To evaluate the effect of local application of ice on duration and severity of acute gouty arthritis.

METHODS:
Nineteen patients with acute gout were enrolled and randomised into two groups. Group A (n = 10) received topical ice therapy, oral prednisone 30 mg PO tapered to 0 over six days and colchicine 0.6 mg/day. Group B was the control group (n = 9), given the same regimen but without the ice therapy. The patients were followed for one week.

RESULTS:
The mean reduction in pain for those patients treated with ice therapy was 7.75 cm (on 10 cm visual analog scale) with standard deviation +/- 2.58 compared with 4.42 cm (+/- SD 2.96) for the control group.

Using a Wilcoxon rank-sum test, there was a significant difference (p = 0.021) in pain reduction between the ice therapy and control groups. Joint circumference and synovial fluid volume also tended to be more effectively reduced after one week of therapy in the ice group compared with controls, but these did not achieve statistical significance.

CONCLUSION:
The group treated with ice had a significantly greater reduction in pain compared with the control group. Although the clinical improvement was impressive, due to the small sample size we could not show statistically significant improvement in all the variables that tended to suggest that effect was more than simply analgesic.

Cold applications may be a useful adjunct to treatment of acute gouty arthritis.

FICTION: Gout attacks come and go and do not cause continuous pain.

FACT: Whilst you may not suffer continuous pain, you still have gout. This is because your uric acid levels don't drop significantly without action (usually in the form of medication), and in the longer term suitable lifestyle changes.

THE BOTTOM LINE: Nurses can be highly effective at helping patients understand gout and as a result to achieve better control of their condition.

Rees F, Jenkins W, Doherty M. Patients with gout adhere to curative treatment if informed appropriately: proof-of-concept observational study. Ann Rheum Dis2013;72:826-30.

Abstract

INTRODUCTION:
Many doctors believe that patients with gout are unwilling to receive urate-lowering therapy (ULT) and blame them for poor adherence to management.

OBJECTIVE:
To test the effectiveness of a complex intervention for gout that incorporates key elements of current guidelines, including full patient information, delivered in an optimal setting (specialist hospital clinic).

METHOD:
Observational study of patients reporting ongoing attacks of gout recruited from primary care lists. 106 participants (94 men, 12 women; mean age 61 years) were enrolled in the study. Patients received a predominantly nurse-delivered intervention that included education, individualised lifestyle advice and appropriate ULT. The predefined goal was to achieve serum uric acid (SUA) levels≤360 µmol/l after one year in at least 70% of participants.

RESULTS:
Of the 106 participants at baseline, 16% had tophi; mean (SD) baseline SUA was 456 (98) µmol/l. All participants agreed to joint aspiration to confirm gout and all wished to receive ULT.

At 12 months, 92% of the 106 participants had achieved the therapeutic target (SUA≤360 µmol); 85% had SUA<300 µmol/l. Allopurinol was the most commonly used ULT, requiring a median dose of 400 mg daily to achieve the target. Improvements in Short Form-36 were observed (significant for pain) after one year.

CONCLUSION:

A predominantly nurse-led intervention including education, lifestyle advice and ULT can successfully achieve the recommended treatment target in more than 9 out of 10 patients. Full explanation and discussion about the nature of gout and its treatment options and individualisation of management probably account for this success.

FICTION: Eating lots of cherries, or drinking cherry concentrate solutions, can cure gout.

FACT: Whatever anyone tells you or claims, there is as yet no cure for gout, and the condition requires lifelong management to relieve and prevent attacks. Even so, there is some evidence to suggest that consuming cherries or medically-approved cherry concentrates could lower your body's uric acid levels, and by implication lower the risk of gout attacks.

THE BOTTOM LINE: Weight loss and calorie intake reduction help reduce high blood uric acid and cholesterol levels.

Dessein PH, Shipton EA, Stanwix AE, Joffe BI, Ramokgadi J. Beneficial effects of weight loss associated with moderate calorie/carbohydrate restriction, and increased proportional intake of protein and unsaturated fat on serum urate and lipoprotein levels in gout: a pilot study. Ann Rheum Dis2000;59:539-43.

Abstract

OBJECTIVES:
Insulin resistance (IR) has been increasingly implicated in the pathogenesis of gout. The lipoprotein abnormalities described in hyperuricaemic subjects are similar to those associated with IR, and insulin influences renal urate excretion.

In this study, it was investigated whether dietary measures, reported to be beneficial in IR, have serum uric acid (SU) and lipid lowering effects in gout.

METHODS:
Thirteen non-diabetic men (median age 50, range 38-62) were enrolled. Each patient had at least two gouty attacks during the four months before enrolment. Dietary recommendations consisted of calorie restriction to 6690 kJ (1600 kcal) a day with 40% derived from carbohydrate, 30% from protein, and 30% from fat; replacement of refined carbohydrates with complex ones and saturated fats with mono- and polyunsaturated ones. At onset and after 16 weeks, fasting blood samples were taken for determination of SU, serum cholesterol (C), low density lipoprotein cholesterol (LDL-C), high density lipoprotein cholesterol (HDL-C), and triglycerides (TGs). Results were expressed as median (SD).

RESULTS:
At onset, the body mass index (BMI) was 30.5 (8.1) kg/m(2). Dietary measures resulted in weight loss of 7.7 (5.4) kg (p=0.002) and a

decrease in the frequency of monthly attacks from 2.1 (0.8) to 0.6 (0.7) (p=0.002).

The SU decreased from 0.57 (0.10) to 0.47 (0.09) mmol/l (p=0.001) and normalised in 7 (58%) of the 12 patients with an initially raised level. Serum cholesterol decreased from 6.0 (1.7) to 4.7 (0. 9) mmol/l (p=0.002), LDL-C from 3.5 (1.2) to 2.7 (0.8) mmol/l (p=0. 004), TGs from 4.7 (4.2) to 1.9 (1.0) mmol/l (p=0.001), and C:HDL-C ratios from 6.7 (1.7) to 5.2 (1.0) (p=0.002). HDL-C levels increased insignificantly. High baseline SU, frequency of attacks, total cholesterol, LDL-C and TG levels, and total C:HDL-C ratios correlated with higher decreases in the respective variables upon dietary intervention (p<0.05).

CONCLUSION:
The results suggest that weight reduction associated with a change in proportional macronutrient intake, as recently recommended in IR, is beneficial, reducing the SU levels and dyslipidaemia in gout. Current dietary recommendations for gout may need re-evaluation.

Kullich W, Ulreich A, Klein G. [Changes in uric acid and blood lipids in patients with asymptomatic hyperuricemia treated with diet therapy in a rehabilitation procedure]. Rehabilitation (Stuttg)1989;28:134-7.

THE BOTTOM LINE: Appropriate dietary advice is highly beneficial for gout.

Abstract

More than 300 patients with asymptomatic hyperuricaemia had been included in lipometabolic analysis performed before and after four weeks of a special low-cholesterol, low-triglyceride and low-purine dietetic regimen.

Remarkable in almost the entire hyperuricaemic population (96.7%) had been the presence of serum cholesterol levels of more than 200 mg/dl.

Lipoprotein analysis showed that 87% of the patients had increased LDL- and 69% increased VLDL-levels; HDL-levels were pathologically lowered to below 40mg/dl in 41% of the group. After a four-week rehabilitation programme, all lipometabolic parameters and serum urate concentrations were found to have been significantly reduced by the special diet.

The results therefore are impressive proof of the major health benefits of purposive nutritional behaviour.

THE BOTTOM LINE: Starting allopurinol during an acute attack of gout is of little benefit.

Taylor TH, Mecchella JN, Larson RJ, Kerin K, MacKenzie TA. Initiation of allopurinol at first medical contact for acute attacks of gout: a randomized clinical trial. Am J Med2012;125:1126-3e7.

Abstract

OBJECTIVE:
Streamlining the initiation of allopurinol could result in a cost benefit for a common medical problem and obviate the perception that no treatment is required once acute attacks have resolved. Our objective was to test the hypothesis that there is no difference in patient daily pain or subsequent attacks with early versus delayed initiation of allopurinol for an acute gout attack.

METHODS:
A total of 57 men with crystal-proven gout were randomised to allopurinol 300 mg daily or matching placebo for 10 days. All subjects received indomethacin 50 mg 3 times per day for 10 days, a prophylactic dose of colchicine 0.6 mg 2 times per day for 90 days, and open-label allopurinol starting at day 11. Primary outcome measures were pain on visual analogue scale (VAS) for the primary joint on days 1 to 10 and self-reported flares in any joint through day 30.

RESULTS:
On the basis of 51 evaluable subjects (allopurinol in 26, placebo in 25), mean daily VAS pain scores did not differ significantly between study groups at any point between days 1 and 10.

Initial VAS pain scores for allopurinol and placebo arms were 6.72 versus 6.28 (P=.37), declining to 0.18 versus 0.27 (P=.54) at day 10, with neither group consistently having more daily pain.

Subsequent flares occurred in two subjects taking allopurinol and three subjects taking placebo (P=.60). Although urate levels decreased rapidly in the allopurinol group (from 7.8 mg/dL at baseline to 5.9 mg/dL at day 3), sedimentation rates and C-reactive protein levels did not differ between groups at any point.

CONCLUSIONS:
Allopurinol initiation during an acute gout attack caused no significant difference in daily pain, recurrent flares, or inflammatory markers.

FICTION: Taking aspirin is a known pain-reliever, and is just as effective for ending gout attacks as ending headaches.

FACT: The opposite is true, because taking aspirin during a gout attack makes it much worse.

THE BOTTOM LINE: Keeping blood levels of uric acid low helps to reduce the amount of urate crystals in joints.

Li-Yu J, Clayburne G, Sieck M, Beutler A, Rull M, Eisner E, et al. Treatment of chronic gout. Can we determine when urate stores are depleted enough to prevent attacks of gout? J Rheumatol 2001;28:577-80.

Abstract

OBJECTIVE:
To determine if lowering of serum uric acid (SUA) concentrations below 6 mg/dl or longer duration of lowered SUA will result in depletion of urate crystals from the knee joints and prevent further attacks of gout.

METHODS:
A prospective study was initiated 10 years ago at Philadelphia VA Medical Center to attempt to maintain SUA levels of patients with crystal proven gout at < 6.0 mg/dl. We recalled all 57 patients who were available during 1999. Patients were divided into two groups: Group A, with SUA still > 6 mg/dl, and Group B, with SUA < or = 6 mg/dl. A knee joint aspirate was requested from all asymptomatic Group B patients and many in Group A. Aspirates were examined by polarised light microscopy for identification of crystals.

RESULTS:
There were no differences between the groups in age, sex, duration of gout, or serum creatinine. Group A (n = 38) had a mean of six attacks of gout for the recent year, those with tophi having the most frequent attacks. Among the 16 patients in this group who agreed to knee aspiration, monosodium urate (MSU) crystals were found in 14, although they were asymptomatic at the time.

Nineteen patients (Group B) were able to maintain serum urate levels < or = 6 mg/dl for > 12 months. Nearly half of them had no attack of gout for two or more years, with a mean of one attack in the last year for the whole group.

Three patients in whom tophi were found did not have major flares of gout within the past year. Knee joint aspiration was done on 16 asymptomatic patients. Seven (44%) still had MSU crystals present in their knees.

Patients in this group who were taking prophylactic colchicine did not differ with respect to the character of synovial fluid from those who had discontinued it for up to several years, although the frequency of attacks was less in those who continued colchicine.

CONCLUSION:
A majority of patients were able to deplete urate crystal stores in their knee joint fluids when their SUA levels were kept to < or = 6 mg/dl for several years. The mechanisms for persistence in some patients, and whether such crystals have clinical implications, are not known. Patients with chronic gout need serum urate concentrations to be kept low to prevent further attacks.

Shoji A, Yamanaka H, Kamatani N. A retrospective study of the relationship between serum urate level and recurrent attacks of gouty arthritis: evidence for reduction of recurrent gouty arthritis with antihyperuricemic therapy. Arthritis Rheum2004;51:321-5.

THE BOTTOM LINE: Similar to the previous research, reducing blood levels of uric acid helps prevent further attacks of gout.

Abstract

OBJECTIVE:
To evaluate the proposed relationship between persistent reduction of serum urate into the subsaturating range and reduction in the frequency of acute gouty attacks.

METHODS:
We retrospectively examined data derived from 267 patients who had experienced at least one gouty attack before their first visit to our clinic. Serum urate concentration, history of recurrent gouty attacks, and information about antihyperuricemic drug use were collected on each visit for up to three years from the first visit of each patient. Data derived from visits >1 year after study entry were subjected to statistical analysis.

RESULTS:
When adjusted for baseline serum urate level and the number of gouty attacks prior to study entry, reduction of follow-up serum urate concentration and antihyperuricemic drug use were each significantly associated with a reduced risk of gouty attacks (odds ratio [OR] 0.42, 95% confidence interval [95% CI] 0.31-0.57; OR 0.22, 95% CI 0.10-0.47, respectively).

CONCLUSION:
The data indicate that reduction of serum urate concentrations to 6 mg/dl or lower will eventually result in a reduced frequency or prevention of future gouty attacks.

THE BOTTOM LINE: Blood levels of uric acid must be low enough to promote the dissolving of uric acid crystals, and allopurinol and benzbromarone are equally effective for this. In some patients, it may be necessary to treat with both drugs.

Perez-Ruiz F, Calabozo M, Pijoan JI, Herrero-Beites AM, Ruibal A. Effect of urate-lowering therapy on the velocity of size reduction of tophi in chronic gout. Arthritis Rheum 2002;47:356-60.

Abstract

OBJECTIVE:
The optimal serum urate levels necessary for elimination of tissue deposits of monosodium urate in patients with chronic gout is controversial. This observational, prospective study evaluates the relationship between serum urate levels during therapy and the velocity of reduction of tophi in patients with chronic tophaceous gout.

METHOD:
Sixty-three patients with crystal-confirmed tophaceous gout were treated with allopurinol, benzbromarone, or combined therapy to achieve serum uric acid levels less than the threshold for saturation of urate in tissues. The tophi targeted for evaluation during follow-up were the largest in diameter found during physical examination.

RESULTS:
Patients taking benzbromarone alone or combined allopurinol and benzbromarone therapy achieved faster velocity of reduction of tophi than patients taking allopurinol alone. The velocity of tophi reduction was linearly related to the mean serum urate level during therapy. The lower the serum urate levels, the faster the velocity of tophi reduction.

CONCLUSION:
Serum urate levels should be lowered enough to promote dissolution of urate deposits in patients with tophaceous gout.

Allopurinol and benzbromarone are equally effective when optimal serum urate levels are achieved during therapy.

Combined therapy may be useful in patients who do not show enough reduction in serum urate levels with single-drug therapy.

FICTION:The incidence of gout in the UK is a media fabrication, and there are very few actual sufferers.

FACT: Gout has become the number one type of inflammatory arthritis in the UK. In fact, according to Arthritis Care:

"Gout affects one in 40 people in the UK. 1 Since 1997 there has been a 30% increase in the number diagnosed with gout, and this statistic continues to increase by 1.5% every year."

THE BOTTOM LINE: This paper emphasises the importance of allopurinol in lowering blood levels of uric acid. The paper also considers its severe side effect risk.

Stamp LK, Taylor WJ, Jones PB, Dockerty JL, Drake J, Frampton C, et al. Starting dose is a risk factor for allopurinol hypersensitivity syndrome: a proposed safe starting dose of allopurinol. Arthritis Rheum2012;64:2529-36. CrossRefMedlineWeb of Science

Dalbeth N, Stamp L. Allopurinol dosing in renal impairment: walking the tight-rope between adequate urate-lowering and adverse events. Semin Dial2007;20:391-5.

Abstract

Allopurinol is the mainstay of urate-lowering therapy for patients with gout and impaired renal function.

Although rare, a life-threatening hypersensitivity syndrome may occur with this drug. The risk of this allopurinol hypersensitivity syndrome (AHS) is increased in renal impairment.

The recognition that AHS may be because of delayed-type hypersensitivity to oxypurinol, the main metabolite of allopurinol, and that oxypurinol concentrations are frequently elevated in patients with renal impairment prescribed standard doses of allopurinol has led to the widespread adoption of allopurinol-dosing guidelines.

These guidelines advocate allopurinol dose reduction according to creatinine clearance in patients with renal impairment. However, recent studies have challenged the role of these guidelines, suggesting that AHS may occur even at low doses of allopurinol, and that these guidelines lead to under-treatment of hyperuricemia, a key therapeutic target in gout.

Based on current data, we advocate gradual introduction of allopurinol according to current treatment guidelines, with close monitoring of serum uric acid concentrations.

In patients with severe disease and persistent hyperuricemia, allopurinol dose escalation above those recommended by the guidelines should be considered, with careful evaluation of the benefits and risks of therapy. Further work is needed to clarify the safety and efficacy of allopurinol dose escalation, particularly in patients with renal impairment.

FICTION: Gout is fully justified in being known as 'the rich man's disease'.

FACT: Although historically linked to the wealthy, gout now affects more people suffering from poverty.

THE BOTTOM LINE: According to this study, vitamin C supplements are of no benefit in helping to lower blood uric acid levels.

Borstad GC, Bryant LR, Abel MP, Scroggie DA, Harris MD, Alloway JA. Colchicine for prophylaxis of acute flares when initiating allopurinol for chronic gouty arthritis. J Rheumatol 2004;31:2429-32.

Tayar JH, Lopez-Olivo MA, Suarez-Almazor ME. Febuxostat for treating chronic gout. Cochrane Database Syst Rev2012;11:CD008653.

National Institute for Health and Care Excellence. Febuxostat for the management of hyperuricaemia in people with gout. TA164. 2011. www.nice.org.uk/nicemedia/live/12101/42738/42738.pdf.

Stamp LK, O'Donnell JL, Frampton C, Drake JM, Zhang M, Chapman PT. Clinically insignificant effect of supplemental vitamin C on serum urate in patients with gout: a pilot randomized controlled trial. Arthritis Rheum. 2013 Jun;65(6):1636-42. doi: 10.1002/art.37925.

Abstract

OBJECTIVE:
Studies in human volunteers have shown that vitamin C reduces serum urate (SU) levels. The aim of this study was to determine the effects of vitamin C on SU levels in patients with gout.

METHODS:
Patients with gout and an SU level >0.36 mmoles/liter (6 mg/dl) were recruited. Twenty patients already taking allopurinol were randomised to receive an increase in the dose of allopurinol or to commence taking vitamin C (500 mg/day). Twenty patients who had not been taking allopurinol were randomised to start receiving either allopurinol (up to 100 mg/day) or vitamin C (500 mg/day). Levels of plasma ascorbate, creatinine, and SU were measured on day 0 and week 8.

RESULTS:

There was no significant difference in the baseline SU level or estimated glomerular filtration rate (eGFR) between those who received vitamin C and those who did not (for SU, mean ± SEM 0.50 ± 0.11 mmoles/liter [8.4 ± 1.8 mg/dl] versus 0.50 ± 0.09 mmoles/liter [8.4 ± 1.5 mg/dl]; for eGFR, mean ± SEM 65.5 ± 3.5 ml/minute/1.73 m(2) versus 67.9 ± 4.6 ml/minute/1.73 m(2)). Among the randomised patients, 30% in the vitamin C group and 25% in the no vitamin C control group were receiving diuretics. In the patients receiving vitamin C, there was a significant increase between day 0 and week 8 in the plasma ascorbate level. The reduction in SU level over 8 weeks was significantly less in those patients receiving vitamin C compared to those who started or increased the dose of allopurinol (mean reduction 0.014 mmoles/liter [0.23 mg/dl] versus 0.118 mmoles/liter [1.9 mg/dl]; P < 0.001).

CONCLUSION:

A modest dosage of vitamin C (500 mg/day) for eight weeks had no clinically significant urate-lowering effects in patients with gout, despite the fact that plasma ascorbate levels increased. These results differ from previous findings in healthy control subjects with hyperuricemia. The uricosuric effect of modest-dose vitamin C appears to be small in patients with gout, when administered as monotherapy or in combination with allopurinol.

The conclusion of the study above is in complete contrast to that of the following study.

THE BOTTOM LINE: In contrast to the previous study, this research shows that vitamin C supplements ARE beneficial in lowering the risk of gout.

Choi HK, Gao X, Curhan G. Vitamin C intake and the risk of gout in men: a prospective study. Arch Intern Med. 2009;169(5):502-7.

Abstract

BACKGROUND:
Several metabolic studies and a recent double-blind, placebo-controlled, randomised trial have shown that higher vitamin C intake significantly reduces serum uric acid levels. Yet the relation with risk of gout is unknown.

METHODS:
We prospectively examined, from 1986 through 2006, the relation between vitamin C intake and risk of incident gout in 46,994 male participants with no history of gout at baseline. We used a supplementary questionnaire to ascertain the American College of Rheumatology criteria for gout. Vitamin C intake was assessed every four years through validated questionnaires.

RESULTS:
During the 20 years of follow-up, we documented 1,317 confirmed incident cases of gout.

Compared with men with vitamin C intake less than 250 mg/d, the multivariate relative risk (RR) of gout was 0.83 (95% confidence interval [CI], 0.71-0.97) for total vitamin C intake of 500 to 999 mg/d, 0.66 (0.52-0.86) for 1000 to 1499 mg/d, and 0.55 (0.38-0.80) for 1500 mg/d or greater (P < .001 for trend).

The multivariate RR per 500-mg increase in total daily vitamin C intake was 0.83 (95% CI, 0.77-0.90). Compared with men who did not use supplemental vitamin C, the multivariate RR of gout was 0.66 (95% CI, 0.49-0.88) for supplemental vitamin C intake of 1000 to 1499 mg/d and 0.55 (0.36-0.86) for 1500 mg/d or greater (P < .001 for trend).

CONCLUSIONS:

Higher vitamin C intake is independently associated with a lower risk of gout.

Supplemental vitamin C intake may be beneficial in the prevention of gout.

FICTION: Whilst gout is quite painful, you can still go about your daily business more or less as usual.

FACT: Not true. In fact, gout severely impacts on day-to-day life. When gout is at its worst, 83% of people have reported struggling with day-to-day activities such as walking. 9% have also reported having to take time off work due to their gout.

SOURCE: Arthritis Care

THE BOTTOM LINE: This paper looks at how lifestyle and dietary recommendations are important in the management of gout and its commonly associated diseases.

Choi HK. A prescription for lifestyle change in patients with hyperuricemia and gout. [Review]. Curr Opin Rheumatol. 2010;22(2):165-72.

Abstract

PURPOSE OF REVIEW:
This review summarises the recent data on lifestyle factors that influence serum uric acid levels and the risk of gout and attempts to provide holistic recommendations, considering both their impact on gout as well as on other health implications.

RECENT FINDINGS:
Large-scale studies have clarified a number of long-suspected relations between lifestyle factors, hyperuricemia, and gout, including purine-rich foods, dairy foods, various beverages, fructose, and vitamin C supplementation. Furthermore, recent studies have identified the substantial burden of comorbidities among patients with hyperuricemia and gout.

SUMMARY:
Lifestyle and dietary recommendations for gout patients should consider overall health benefits and risk, since gout is often associated with the metabolic syndrome and an increased future risk of cardiovascular disease (CVD) and mortality.

Weight reduction with daily exercise and limiting intake of red meat and sugary beverages would help reduce uric acid levels, the risk of gout, insulin resistance, and comorbidities.

Heavy drinking should be avoided, whereas moderate drinking, sweet fruits, and seafood intake, particularly oily fish, should be tailored to the individual, considering their anticipated health benefits against CVD.

Dairy products, vegetables, nuts, legumes, fruits (less sugary ones), and wholegrains are healthy choices for the comorbidities of gout and may also help prevent gout by reducing insulin resistance.

Coffee and vitamin C supplementation could be considered as preventive measures as these can lower urate levels, as well as the risk of gout and some of its comorbidities.

FICTION: Gout attacks you physically, but it doesn't make you feel depressed.

FACT: Suffering a gout attack has a major effect on someone's mental health (as well as physical) with over a third of people feeling depressed during a gout attack.

THE BOTTOM LINE: Recent research emphasises the links between dietary and other factors and the risk for gout.

Choi HK. Diet, alcohol, and gout: how do we advise patients given recent developments? Curr RheumatolRep. 2005;7(3):220-6.

Abstract

The disease burden of gout remains substantial and may be increasing as a result of trends in demographics and lifestyles.

Recent scientific data serve to illuminate the links between dietary and other factors and risk for gout.

These lifestyle factors affect not only the risk for gout, but are also risk factors for other chronic diseases of public health importance.

Accordingly, dietary and lifestyle recommendations related to gout should consider their effect on many diseases beyond gout.

These recommendations should ideally reinforce the established recommendations where the influence on gout parallels the influence on other diseases, and consider modifying the recommendations where they are divergent.

THE BOTTOM LINE: Coffee seems to help reduce the risk of gout (particularly for women)

Choi HK, Curhan G. Coffee consumption and risk of incident gout in women: the Nurses' Health Study. Am J Clin Nutr. 2010;92(4):922-7.

Abstract

BACKGROUND:
Coffee is one of the most widely consumed beverages in the world and may affect the risk of gout via various mechanisms, but prospective data on the relation between coffee intake and the risk of incident gout are limited.

DESIGN:
Over a 26-year period, we prospectively examined the relation between coffee intake and risk of incident gout in 89,433 female participants in the Nurses' Health Study. We assessed the consumption of coffee, decaffeinated coffee, tea, and total caffeine in participants every two to four years through validated questionnaires.

We used a supplementary questionnaire to ascertain whether participants met the survey criteria of the American College of Rheumatology for gout. Results: During the 26 years of follow-up, we documented 896 confirmed incident cases of gout.

There was an inverse association between higher coffee intake and the risk of gout.

The multivariate relative risks (RRs) for incident gout according to coffee-consumption categories [ie, 0, 1-237, 238-947, and ≥948 mL coffee/d (237 mL = one 8-ounce cup)] were 1.00, 0.97, 0.78 (95% CI: 0.64, 0.95), and 0.43 (95% CI: 0.30, 0.61; P for trend < 0.0001), respectively. For decaffeinated coffee, the multivariate RRs according to consumption categories (0, 1-237, and ≥237 mL decaffeinated coffee/d) were 1.00, 1.02, and 0.77 (95% CI: 0.63, 0.95; P for trend = 0.02), respectively.

There was an inverse association between total caffeine from all sources and the risk of gout; the multivariate RR of the highest quintile compared with the lowest quintile was 0.52 (95% CI: 0.41, 0.68; P for trend <0.0001).

CONCLUSION:

These prospective data suggest that long-term coffee consumption is associated with a lower risk of incident gout in women.

FICTION: Gout can only be caused by 'external' factors, such as diet and lifestyle.

FACT: Whilst gout attacks are often more frequent due to factors such as poor diet and being overweight or obese, about one in five gout causes are due to hereditary reasons.

THE BOTTOM LINE: This paper looks at several new strategies for the treatment of gout.

Dubchak N, Falasca GF. New and improved strategies for the treatment of gout. Int J Nephrol Renovasc Dis. 2010;3:145-66.

Abstract

The Western world appears to be in the midst of the third great gout epidemic of all time.

In this century, gout is increasing in prevalence despite an increased understanding of its risk factors and pathophysiology, and the availability of reasonably effective treatment.

The main cultural factors responsible for this appear to be diet, obesity, ethanol use and medications.

Excess fructose consumption is a newly recognised modifiable risk factor.

The debate has been renewed concerning hyperuricemia as an independent risk factor for renal insufficiency and cardiovascular disease. Prevention is still rooted in lifestyle choices.

Existing treatments have proven to be unsatisfactory in many patients with comorbidities.

New treatments are available today and on the horizon for tomorrow, which offer a better quality of life for gout sufferers.

These include febuxostat, a nonpurine inhibitor of xanthine oxidase with a potentially better combination of efficacy and safety than allopurinol, and investigational inhibitors of URAT-1, an anion exchanger in the proximal tubule that is critical for uric acid homeostasis.

New abortive treatments include interleukin-1 antagonists that can cut short the acute attack in one to two days in persons who cannot take nonsteroidal anti-inflammatory drugs, colchicine or corticosteroids.

Lastly, newer formulations of uricase have the ability to dissolve destructive tophi over weeks or months in patients who cannot use currently available hypouricemic agents.

Diagnostically, ultrasound and magnetic resonance imaging offer advanced ways to diagnose gout noninvasively, and just as importantly, a way to follow the progress of tophus dissolution.

The close association of hyperuricemia with metabolic syndrome, hypertension and renal insufficiency ensures that nephrologists will see increasing numbers of gout-afflicted patients.

THE BOTTOM LINE: Although the most effective dietary advice for gout is yet to be fully established, the current advice is to consume meat, seafood and alcohol in moderation and to be careful about portion size and the consumption of high GI carbs in order to help weight loss and insulin sensitivity.

Eggebeen AT. Gout: an update. Am Fam Physician. 2007;76(6):801-8. Review.

Falasca GF. Metabolic diseases: gout. Clin Dermatol. 2006;24(6):498-508.

Hak AE, Choi HK. Lifestyle and Gout. Curr Opin Rheumatol. 2008;20(2):179-86.

Jana S, Shekhawat GS. Critical review on medicinally potent plant species: Gloriosa superba. [Review]. Fitoterapia. 2011;82(3):293-301.

Kang EH, Lee EY, Lee YJ, Song YW, Lee EB. Clinical features and risk factors of postsurgical gout. Ann Rheum Dis. 2008;67(9):1271-5.

Lee SJ, Terkeltaub RA, Kavanaugh A. Recent developments in diet and gout. Curr Opin Rheumatol. 2006;18(2):193-8.

Abstract

PURPOSE OF REVIEW:
Gout is the most common inflammatory arthritis in men, affecting approximately 1-2% of adult men in Western countries. United States gout prevalence has approximately doubled over the past two decades.

In recent years, key prospective epidemiological and open-labeled dietary studies, coupled with recent advances in molecular biology elucidating proximal tubular urate transport, have provided novel insights into roles of diet and alcohol in hyperuricemia and gout. This review focuses on recent developments and their implications for clinical practice, including how we advise patients on appropriate diets and alcoholic beverage consumption.

RECENT FINDINGS:
Studies have observed an increased risk of gout among those who consumed the highest quintile (i.e. the top 20% of consumers) of meat, seafood and alcohol. Although limited by confounding variables, low-fat dairy products, ascorbic acid and wine consumption appeared to be protective for the development of gout.

SUMMARY:
The most effective forms of dietary regimen for both hyperuricemia and gout flares remains to be unidentified. Until confirmed by a large, controlled study, it is prudent to advise patients to consume meat, seafood and alcoholic beverages in moderation, with special attention to food portion size and content of non-complex carbohydrates which are essential for weight loss and improved insulin sensitivity.

THE BOTTOM LINE: The most effective way to manage gout is by understanding its causes, prevention and drug treatments.

Li EK. Gout: a review of its aetiology and treatment. Hong Kong Med J. 2004;10(4):261-70.

Abstract

OBJECTIVE:
To review the current understanding of the causes and the management of gout.

DATA SOURCES:
Publications on all peer-review literature from MEDLINE from 1965 to January 2004.

STUDY SELECTION:
Selected and evaluated by the author.

DATA EXTRACTION:
Extracted and evaluated by the author.

DATA SYNTHESIS:
The underlying metabolic disorder in gout is hyperuricaemia.

Most patients with hyperuricaemia remain asymptomatic throughout their lifetime. The phase of asymptomatic hyperuricaemia ends with the first attack of gouty arthritis or urolithiasis.

The risk of gout and stone formation is increased with the degree and duration of hyperuricaemia.

Drugs available for the treatment of acute gouty arthritis, such as non-steroidal anti-inflammatory drugs, selective cyclo-oxygenase 2 inhibitors, systemic corticosteroids, or colchicine, are effective.

For periods between attacks, prophylactic therapy, such as low-dose colchicine, is effective. In those with recurrent attacks of more than two to three times yearly, a uric acid-lowering agent as a long-term therapy should be considered to avoid recurrence and the development of tophaceous gout.

CONCLUSIONS:

Effective management of gout can be achieved through better understanding of the causes of the condition, preventive measures as well as drug treatment.

FICTION: Eating protein causes gout attacks.

FACT: Yes and no. Certain types of meat have been shown to raise uric acid levels. However, the proteins in broccoli, Brussels sprouts, peas and spinach provide you with protein and actually lower uric acid levels.

THE BOTTOM LINE: Good gout management depends on a proper diagnosis based on finding uric acid crystals, a clear aim to eliminate crystals from joints and elsewhere, the use of alternative medications if necessary, and promoting a healthy lifestyle.

Li S, Micheletti R. Role of diet in rheumatic disease. [Review]. Rheum Dis Clin North Am. 2011;37(1):119-33.

Pascual E, Sivera F. Therapeutic advances in gout. Curr Opin Rheumatol. 2007;19(2):122-7.

Abstract

PURPOSE OF REVIEW:
The purpose of this review is to highlight the recent developments in the management of gout.

RECENT FINDINGS:
Guidelines for the diagnosis and management of gout from EULAR, quality of care indicators, and outcome measures for clinical trials have been published. The standards of gout diagnosis and management are very low.

Allopurinol remains the mainstay for serum uric acid lowering therapy. In an important percentage of patients receiving allopurinol, serum uric acid levels are insufficient to promote crystal dissolution.

Febuxostat, a new serum uric acid lowering drug, has shown good results. Information on uricase continues to appear.

For treatment of gouty inflammation, etoricoxib (a new cyclooxygenase 2 inhibitor) has been shown to be as effective as indomethacin.

Finally, the association of gout with the metabolic syndrome and its comorbidities, and the newly described association of gout with myocardial infarction, bring lifestyle and dietary modifications to the front in the management of gout.

SUMMARY:

Proper gout management requires changes to the physician's attitude towards the disease; essentially:

1. an unequivocal diagnosis based in urate crystal identification,

2. a clearly settled aim of the treatment: crystal elimination from the joints and elsewhere, and

3. proper use of the available therapeutic alternatives. Promoting a proper lifestyle appears to be especially important.

Goutbusters Tip #1

Make sure you really do have gout –and not another condition. Book an appointment and tests with your doctor if you're not certain.

Go to page 179 for the next tip...

THE BOTTOM LINE: This paper highlights the importance of early identification of patients with high blood levels of uric acid.

Peterson DM. Nonsteroidal anti-inflammatory drugs and colchicine to prevent gout flare during early urate-lowering therapy: perspectives on alternative therapies and costs. J Pain

Palliat Care Pharmacother. 2010;24(4):402-4.

Rakel & Bope: Conn's Current Therapy 2009, 1st ed. Philadelphia, PA: Saunders Elsevier. 2008.

Richette P, Bardin T. Gout. Lancet. 2010;375(9711):318-28.

Saag KG, Choi H. Epidemiology, risk factors, and lifestyle modifications for gout. ArthritisRes Ther. 2006;8 Suppl 1:S2.

Abstract

Gout affects more than 1% of adults in the USA, and it is the most common form of inflammatory arthritis among men. Accumulating data support an increase in the prevalence of gout that is potentially attributable to recent shifts in diet and lifestyle, improved medical care, and increased longevity.

There are both nonmodifiable and modifiable risk factors for hyperuricemia and gout.

Nonmodifiable risk factors include age and sex.

Gout prevalence increases in direct association with age; the increased longevity of populations in industrialised nations may contribute to a higher prevalence of gout through the disorder's association with aging-related diseases such as metabolic syndrome and hypertension, and treatments for these diseases such as thiazide diuretics for hypertension.

Although gout is considered to be primarily a male disease, there is a more equal sex distribution among elderly patients.

Modifiable risk factors for gout include obesity, the use of certain medications, high purine intake, and consumption of purine-rich alcoholic beverages.

The increasing prevalence of gout worldwide indicates that there is an urgent need for improved efforts to identify patients with hyperuricemia early in the disease process, before the clinical manifestations of gout become apparent.

Goutbusters Tip #2

Once you know for sure you have gout, it's time to prepare your **Goutbusters Action Plan**, and focus on the key areas for reducing both the duration and intensity of gout attacks, and relieving your pain when they do strike.

Go to page 184 for the next tip...

THE BOTTOM LINE: This paper looks at recent developments in the drug treatment of gout.

Schelesinger N. Overview of the management of acute gout and the role of adrenocorticotropic hormone. Drugs. 2008; 68(4):407-15.

Schlesinger N, Dalbeth N, Perez-Ruiz F. Gout - what are the treatment options? Expert Opin Pharmacother. 2009;10(8):1319-28.

Abstract

There has been an increase in the incidence and prevalence of gout in the past several decades.

A distinction needs to be made between the treatment of gout as an acute inflammatory disease and the lowering of the serum urate (SU) levels into a normal range.

Treating acute gout attacks alone is not sufficient to prevent the disease from progressing. When treating gout one needs to treat acute attacks, and lower excess stores of uric acid to achieve dissolution of monosodium urate crystals through a long-term reduction of SU concentrations far beyond the threshold for saturation of urate and provide prophylaxis to prevent acute flares.

The options available for the treatment of acute gout are NSAIDs, colchicine, corticosteroids, adrenocorticotropic hormone (ACTH) and intra-articular corticosteroids.

The most important determinant of therapeutic success is not which anti-inflammatory agent is chosen, but rather how soon therapy is initiated and that the dose be appropriate. Prophylaxis should be considered an adjunct, rather than an alternative, to long-term urate-lowering therapy. For purposes of maintaining patient adherence to urate-lowering therapy, there is interest in improving prophylaxis of such treatment-induced attacks.

The optimal agent, dose and duration for gout prophylaxis are unknown and require further investigation. The importance of long-term management of gout is the reduction and maintenance of SU in a goal range, usually defined as less than 6.0 mg/dL.

Allopurinol and benzbromarone remain the cornerstone drugs for reducing SU levels lower than the saturation threshold to dissolve urate deposits effectively.

Febuxostat and pegloticase help to optimise control of SU levels, especially in those patients with the most severe gout. Other agents, such as fenofibrate and losartan, may be helpful as adjuvant drugs.

Treatment for gout has advanced little in the last 40 years, until recently. The recent development of new therapeutic options promises to provide much needed alternatives for the many patients with gout who are intolerant of or refractory to available therapies. It is important to note that inappropriate use of medications as opposed to an apparent refractoriness to available therapies is not uncommon.

THE BOTTOM LINE: This is another paper that looks at recent developments in the drug treatment of gout.

Schumacher HR Jr, Chen LX. Newer therapeutic approaches: gout. Rheum Dis Clin North Am. 2006;32(1):235-44, xii. Review.

Abstract

Newer approaches to the treatment of gout have included modifications and further attention to aspects of current therapies, and development of interesting new therapies.

Colchicine prophylaxis appears to be needed longer than previously recognised after introduction of a urate-lowering agent.

Diet has received attention, though most dietary effects are small.

New agents under investigation include pegylated formulations of uricase and a new potent xanthine oxidase inhibitor, febuxostat.

Some cardiovascular drugs have been shown to be uricosuric (i.e. substances that increase the excretion of uric acid in the urine, thus reducing the concentration of uric acid in blood plasma).

THE BOTTOM LINE: This is an interesting and wide-ranging paper.

Not only does it look at recently available drugs, it also suggests that oral corticosteroids are preferable to non-steroidal anti-inflammatory drugs for patients with acute gout – which is not how most doctors treat the condition.

The paper also confirms the importance of diet and, most interestingly, discusses how local ice therapy might help to differentiate gout from other forms of inflammatory arthritis, and that supplementation with vitamin C may help to reduce risk of gout.

All in all, quite a lot of controversial conclusions.

Suresh E, Das P. Recent advances in management of gout. QJM. 2011 Dec 23

Abstract

Incidence and prevalence of gout have markedly increased over the last few decades in keeping with the rise in prevalence of obesity and metabolic syndrome.

Until recently, management of gout in patients with associated metabolic syndrome and comorbid illnesses such as renal impairment was difficult because of limited treatment options.

However, significant progress has been made in the last few years, with introduction of new treatments such as interleukin-1 antagonists for management of acute gout, and febuxostat and pegloticase for chronic gout.

The association of gout with alcohol, dietary purines and fructose ingestion has been confirmed in large prospective studies, thus enabling the clinician to now provide evidence-based advice to patients.

Recent efficacy and safety data favour lower over higher doses of colchicine, and oral corticosteroids over non-steroidal anti-inflammatory drugs for patients with acute gout.

Local ice therapy might help to differentiate gout from other forms of inflammatory arthritis, and supplementation with vitamin C help to reduce risk of gout.

Several other drugs with rational mechanisms of action are in the pipeline, and likely to be introduced over the next few years. A new era has thus begun in the field of gout.

Goutbusters Tip #3

Make a list of all the foods you eat: are you eating too many foods which can lead to more frequent gout attacks? (Refer to the book and your *'Traffic Light Test'* for full details.)

Go to page 186 for the next tip...

THE BOTTOM LINE: Taila prepared from Guduchi was found to have the effect of stimulating the immune system. The formulation prepared with Ghrita exhibited an anti-stress effect and had the effect of suppressing the immune system.

Vaghamshi R, Jaiswal M, Patgiri BJ, Prajapati PK, Ravishankar B, Shukla VJ. A comparative pharmacological evaluation of Taila (oil) and Ghrita (ghee) prepared with Guduchi (Tinospora cordifolia). Ayu. 2010;31(4):504-8.

Abstract

Guduchi (Tinospora cordifolia wild miers) is a well-known medicinal plant, which is abundantly used in different ayurvedic formulations utilising varieties of media.

The drug has properties like Rasayana (rejuvenating property), Krimighna (anthelmintics), and Kushtghna (used in skin disorders), as described in ayurvedic literature. Taila (oil) and Ghrita (ghee) are used as media in Ayurvedic Sneha (oleaginous) formulations.

Both the test drugs, Guduchi Taila and Ghrita, are prescribed in Vatrakta (gout) and also indicated for Kushtha (skin disorder).

With all these details, the Guduchi Taila and Guduchi Ghrita samples, prepared by using Taila and Ghrita as media, have been subjected to comparative pharmacological investigations, to assess the impact of the media on the expression of pharmacological activity.

The formulations have been evaluated for immunomodulation, anti-inflammatory, and anti-stress activities.

Both the formulations have been found to be active in most of the experiments, however, with the change of media, their results vary at different levels.

Taila prepared from Guduchi was found to have an immunostimulating activity. The formulation prepared with Ghrita exhibited an anti-stress effect with an immunosuppressing activity.

Goutbusters Tip #4

You should also increase your intake of gout-busting food groups, such as cruciferous vegetables and dairy products.

Go to page 188 for the next tip...

THE BOTTOM LINE: Devil's claw extract seems effective in the treatment of rheumatic diseases, including gout.

Wegener T, Lupke NP. Treatment of patients with arthrosis of hip or knee with an aqueous extract of devil's claw (Harpagophytum procumbens DC.). Phytother Res 2003;17(10):1165-1172.

Abstract

Preparations made from the secondary tubers of Devil's claw (Harpagophytum procumbens) are successfully used in patients with rheumatic diseases (arthrosis and low back pain).

In order to add data on the efficacy and long-term safety of an aqueous extract (Doloteffin; 2400 mg extract daily, corresponding to 50 mg harpagoside), which has been tested successfully in patients with low back pain, an uncontrolled multicentre drug surveillance study for about 12 weeks was conducted in 75 patients with arthrosis of the hip or knee.

To standardise the assessment of treatment effects, the Western Ontario and McMaster Universities (WOMAC) osteoarthritis index (10 point scale) as well as the 10 cm VAS pain scale were used.

The results of the study revealed a strong reduction of pain and the symptoms of osteoarthritis. There was a relevant improvement of each WOMAC subscale as well as of the total WOMAC index: 23.8% for the pain subscale, 22.2% for the stiffness subscale and 23.1% for the physical function subscale.

The WOMAC total score was reduced by 22.9%. VAS pain scores were decreased by 25.8% for actual pain, 25.2% for average pain, 22.6% for worst pain and 24.5% for the total pain score.

The physicians reported a continuous improvement in typical clinical findings such as 45.5% for pain on palpation, 35% for limitation of mobility and 25.4% for joint crepitus.

Only two cases of possible adverse drug reactions were reported (dyspeptic complaints and a sensation of fullness). Although this was an open clinical study, the results suggest that this Devil's claw extract has a clinically beneficial effect in the treatment of arthrosis of the hip or knee.

Goutbusters Tip #5

If you regularly drink alcohol, then you should cut back – or cut it out altogether. Your joints will thank you for it.

Go to page 194 for the next tip...

THE BOTTOM LINE: The combination of blood-letting cupping and herbal medicine is effective for gout.

Cupping is a technique whereby a localised vacuum applied against the skin breaks superficial blood vessels in a layer of the skin just below the surface.

It is known as wet cupping if the skin is first incised, which results in the actual removal of blood. It is a very popular practice in some countries, especially Korea.

Zhang SJ, Liu JP, He KQ. Treatment of acute gouty arthritis by blood-letting cupping plus herbal medicine. J Tradit Chin Med. 2010;30(1):18-20.

Abstract

OBJECTIVE:
To observe the therapeutic effect of blood-letting cupping plus herbal medicine for acute gouty arthritis.

METHODS:
The 34 cases of acute gouty arthritis were treated by blood-letting cupping plus herbal medicine.

RESULTS:
21 cases were cured and 13 cases improved.

CONCLUSION:
The therapeutic effect of this therapy (i.e. blood-letting) was satisfactory for gouty arthritis.

THE BOTTOM LINE: The removal of iron improves the outcome of gouty arthritis.

Facchini FS. Near-iron deficiency-induced remission of gouty arthritis. Rheumatology (Oxford). 2003 Dec;42(12):1550-5. Epub 2003 Jun 27.

Abstract

OBJECTIVES:
Previous evidence supports a role for iron in the pathogenesis of gout. For example, iron, when added to media containing urate crystals, stimulated oxidative stress with subsequent complement and neutrophil activation. Conversely, iron removal inhibited these responses as well as urate-crystal-induced footpad inflammation in rats in-vivo. The objective of the present study was to investigate whether or not iron removal may improve the outcome of gouty arthritis in humans as well.

METHODS:
Quantitative phlebotomy was used to remove iron in 12 hyperuricaemic patients with gouty arthritis and maintain their body iron at near-iron deficiency (NID) level (i.e. the lowest body iron store compatible with normal erythropoiesis and therefore absence of anaemia).

RESULTS:
During maintenance of NID for 28 months, gouty attacks markedly diminished in every patient, from a cumulative amount of 48 and 53 attacks per year before (year -2, -1), to 32, 11 and 7 during induction (year 0) and maintenance (year +1, +2) of NID, respectively. During NID, attacks were also more often of milder severity.

CONCLUSIONS:
During a 28-month follow-up, maintenance of NID was found to be safe and beneficial in all patients, with effects ranging from a complete remission to a marked reduction of incidence and severity of gouty attacks.

THE BOTTOM LINE: There is an independent association between gout and the formation of kidney stones.

However they share a common mechanism by which they occur, and working out precisely what those mechanisms are would help improve preventive strategies for both conditions.

Krishnan E, Griffith C, Kwoh C. Burden of illness from gout in ambulatory care in the United States. Abstracts of the American College of Rheumatology 69th annual meeting and the Association of Rheumatology Health Professionals 40th annual meeting. November 12–17, 2005, San Diego, Calif. Arthritis Rheum. 2005;52(9 suppl):S656.

Mikuls TR, Farrar JT, Bilker WB, Fernandes S, Saag KG. Suboptimal physician adherence to quality indicators for the management of gout and asymptomatic hyperuricaemia: results from the UK General Practice Research Database (GPRD). Rheumatology (Oxford). 2005;44:1038–42.

Kramer HM, Curhan G. The association between gout and nephrolithiasis: the National Health and Nutrition Examination Survey III, 1988–1994. Am J Kidney Dis. 2002;40:37–42.

Abstract

BACKGROUND:
Gout, an inflammatory arthritis, reportedly afflicts more than two million men and women in the United States.

Previous reports have suggested an association between gout and kidney stone disease; however, these studies did not adjust for such important potential confounders as obesity and the presence of hypertension.

To our knowledge, no published study has examined the independent association between gout and kidney stone disease.

METHODS:
We used a national probability sample of the US population to determine the independent association between reported gout and history of kidney stone disease.

RESULTS:
Among men and women 20 years and older, 5.6% (10 million) reported the previous passage of a kidney stone and 2.7% (5.1 million) reported a diagnosis of gout by a physician.

Moreover, 8.6% of individuals who reported the passage of a kidney stone on two or more occasions had a history of gout.

Conversely, the prevalence of previous kidney stones in subjects with reported gout was 13.9%. In the age-adjusted model, gout was associated with an increased odds ratio (OR) for previous kidney stones (OR, 1.97; 95% confidence interval [CI], 1.37 to 2.83).

After further adjustment for sex, race, body mass index, and presence of hypertension, the OR for previous kidney stones in individuals with gout decreased to 1.49 (95% CI, 1.04 to 2.14).

CONCLUSION:
Showing an independent association between kidney stone disease and gout strongly suggests that they share common underlying pathophysiological mechanisms. Identification of these mechanisms may lead to improved preventive strategies for both conditions.

THE BOTTOM LINE: The prevalence of gout and/or hyperuricemia (high blood levels of uric acid) have increased over the past few years.

Wallace KL, Riedel AA, Joseph-Ridge N, Wortmann R. Increasing prevalence of gout and hyperuricemia over 10 years among older adults in a managed care population. J Rheumatol. 2004;31:1582–7.

Abstract

OBJECTIVE:
To determine whether the prevalence of gout and/or clinically significant hyperuricemia increased in a managed care population over 10 years.

METHODS:
The study was a descriptive analysis utilising an administrative claims database to ascertain 10-year trends in prevalence of gout and/or hyperuricemia. Prevalence rates were calculated cross-sectionally for each year (1990-99) and expressed/compared as rates per 1000 enrolees.

RESULTS:
The prevalence of gout and/or hyperuricemia in the overall population increased by about two cases per 1000 enrolees over 10 years.

In the > 75 year age group, rates increased from 21 per 1,000 persons in 1990 to 41 per 1,000 in 1999.

In the 65-74 year age group, prevalence increased from between 21 and 24 per 1,000 persons in the years 1990-92 to over 31 per 1,000 during the years 1997-99.

Prevalence rates in younger age groups (< 65 years) stayed consistently low during the years under study. There were sex differences in most age groups, with men having the greater burden of disease at every time point.

CONCLUSION:

Prevalence of gout and/or hyperuricemia in the overall study population increased during the 10-year period.

When stratified by age, there were increases in prevalence among groups over age 65 in both sexes.

Although gout prevalence increased in both sexes over the 10-year period, men still had most of the burden of disease. In ages younger than 65, men had four times higher prevalence than women (4:1 ratio), but in the older age groups (> 65), the gender gap narrowed to one woman to every three men with gout and/or hyperuricemia (3:1 ratio).

Goutbusters Tip #6

Sugar, particularly fructose found in chocolate and sugar, is also another key factor in causing gout pain. Make sure you reduce your sugar intake, or eliminate it altogether from your diet.

Go to page 198 for the next tip...

THE BOTTOM LINE: There was a suggestion that measuring blood uric acid levels might be helpful in predicting coronary heart disease. However this paper suggests that this is unlikely to be so.

Vasan RS, Pencina MJ, Cobain M, Freiberg MS, D'Agostino RB. Estimated risks for developing obesity in the Framingham Heart Study. Ann Intern Med. 2005;143:473–80.

Wu XW, Lee CC, Muzny DM, Caskey CT. Urate oxidase: primary structure and evolutionary implications. Proc Natl Acad Sci USA. 1989;86:9412–6.

Johnson WD, Kayser KL, Brenowitz JB, Saedi SF. A randomized controlled trial of allopurinol in coronary bypass surgery. Am Heart J. 1991;1211 pt 120–4.

Sundstrom J, Sullivan L, D'Agostino RB, Levy D, Kannel WB, Vasan RS. Relations of serum uric acid to longitudinal blood pressure tracking and hypertension incidence. Hypertension. 2005;45:28–33.

Feig DI, Nakagawa T, Karumanchi SA, Oliver WJ, Kang DH, Finch J, et al. Hypothesis: uric acid, nephron number and the pathogenesis of essential hypertension. Kidney Int.2004;66:281–7.

Wheeler JG, Juzwishin KD, Eiriksdottir G, Gudnason V, Danesh J. Serum uric acid and coronary heart disease in 9,458 incident cases and 155,084 controls: prospective study and meta-analysis. PLoS Med. 2005;2:e76.

Abstract

BACKGROUND:

It has been suggested throughout the past 50 years that serum uric acid concentrations can help predict the future risk of coronary heart disease (CHD), but the epidemiological evidence is uncertain.

METHODS AND FINDINGS:

We report a "nested" case-control comparison within a prospective study in Reykjavik, Iceland, using baseline values of serum uric acid in 2,456 incident CHD cases and in 3,962 age- and sex-matched controls, plus paired serum uric acid measurements taken at baseline and, on average, 12 years later in 379 participants. In addition, we conducted a meta-analysis of 15 other prospective studies in eight countries conducted in essentially general populations.

Compared with individuals in the bottom third of baseline measurements of serum uric acid in the Reykjavik study, those in the top third had an age- and sex-adjusted odds ratio for CHD of 1.39 (95% confidence interval [CI], 1.23-1.58) which fell to 1.12 (CI, 0.97-1.30) after adjustment for smoking and other established risk factors.

Overall, in a combined analysis of 9,458 cases and 155,084 controls in all 16 relevant prospective studies, the odds ratio was 1.13 (CI, 1.07-1.20), but it was only 1.02 (CI, 0.91-1.14) in the eight studies with more complete adjustment for possible confounders.

CONCLUSIONS:

Measurement of serum uric acid levels is unlikely to enhance usefully the prediction of CHD, and this factor is unlikely to be a major determinant of the disease in general populations.

THE BOTTOM LINE: This paper seems to contradict the previous paper. (Medicine is rarely clear-cut!) The authors show that gouty arthritis is associated with an excess risk of acute heart attacks.

Krishnan E, Baker JF, Furst DE, Schumacher HR. Gout and the risk of acute myocardial infarction. Arthritis Rheum. 2006;54:2688–96.

Abstract

OBJECTIVE:
To determine if hyperuricemia and gouty arthritis are independent risk factors for acute myocardial infarction (MI) and, if so, whether they are independent of renal function, diuretic use, metabolic syndrome, and other established risk factors.

METHODS:
We performed multivariable logistic and instrumental variable probit regressions on data from the Multiple Risk Factor Intervention Trial (MRFIT).

RESULTS:
Overall, there were 12,866 men in the MRFIT who were followed up for a mean of 6.5 years. There were 118 events of acute MI in the group with gout (10.5%) and 990 events in the group without gout (8.43%; P = 0.018). Hyperuricemia was an independent risk factor for acute MI in the multivariable regression models, with an odds ratio (OR) of 1.11 (95% confidence interval [95% CI] 1.08-1.15, P < 0.001).

In multivariable regressions in which the above risk factors were used as covariates, gout was found to be associated with a higher risk of acute MI (OR 1.26 [95% CI 1.14-1.40], P < 0.001).

Subgroup analyses showed that a relationship between gout and the risk of acute MI was present among non-users of alcohol, diuretics, or aspirin and among those who did not have metabolic syndrome, diabetes mellitus, or obesity. In separate analyses, a relationship between gout and the risk of acute MI was evident among those with and without those hyperuricemia.

CONCLUSION:

The independent risk relationship between hyperuricemia and acute MI is confirmed. Gouty arthritis is associated with an excess risk of acute MI, and this is not explained by its well-known links with renal function, metabolic syndrome, diuretic use, and traditional cardiovascular risk factors.

Goutbusters Tip #7

Do everything you can to lose weight. Being overweight or obese is one of the main causes of increased frequency of gout attacks.

Go to page 201 for the next tip...

THE BOTTOM LINE: The strongest predictors of gout are age, weight, high blood pressure, cholesterol level and alcohol intake.

Campion EW, Glynn RJ, DeLabry LO. Asymptomatic hyperuricemia. Risks and consequences in the Normative Aging Study. Am J Med. 1987;82:421–6.

Abstract

To quantify the consequences of asymptomatic hyperuricemia, this study examined rates for a first episode of gouty arthritis based on 30,147 human-years of prospective observation.

A cohort of 2,046 initially healthy men in the Normative Aging Study was followed for 14.9 years with serial examinations and measurement of urate levels. With prior serum urate levels of 9 mg/dl or more, the annual incidence rate of gouty arthritis was 4.9 percent, compared with 0.5 percent for urate levels of 7.0 to 8.9 mg/dl and 0.1 percent for urate levels below 7.0 mg/dl.

With urate levels of 9 mg/dl or higher, cumulative incidence of gouty arthritis reached 22 percent after five years. Incidence rates were three times higher for hypertensive patients than for normotensive patients (p less than 0.01).

The strongest predictors of gout in a proportional hazards model were age, body mass index, hypertension, and cholesterol level, and alcohol intake.

When the serum urate level became a factor in the model, none of these variables retained independent predictive power. At the final examination, only 0.7 percent of participants had a serum creatinine level of 2.0 mg/dl or more, with no evidence of renal deterioration attributable to hyperuricemia. These data support conservative management of asymptomatic hyperuricemia.

THE BOTTOM LINE: Being overweight and gaining weight are strong risk factors for gout in men, whilst losing weight is protective. High blood pressure and prescribed diuretics are also important risk factors for gout.

Choi HK, Atkinson K, Karlson EW, Curhan G. Obesity, weight change, hypertension, diuretic use, and risk of gout in men: the health professionals follow-up study. Arch Intern Med. 2005;165:742–8.

Abstract

BACKGROUND:
Limited prospective information exists on the relation between obesity and weight change and the risk of gout. Similarly, both hypertension and diuretic use have been considered risk factors for gout; however, their independent contributions have not been established prospectively.

METHODS:
We prospectively examined over a 12-year period (1986-1998) the relation between adiposity, weight change, hypertension, and diuretic use and incident gout in 47,150 male participants with no history of gout at baseline. We used a supplementary questionnaire to ascertain the American College of Rheumatology criteria for gout.

RESULTS:
During 12 years, we documented 730 confirmed incident cases of gout. Compared with men with a body mass index (BMI) of 21 to 22.9, the multivariate relative risks (RRs) of gout were 1.95 (95% confidence interval [CI], 1.44-2.65) for men with a BMI of 25 to 29.9, 2.33 (95% CI, 1.62-3.36) for men with a BMI of 30 to 34.9, and 2.97 (95% CI, 1.73-5.10) for men with a BMI of 35 or greater (P for trend <.001).

Compared with men who had maintained their weight (+/-4 lb) since age 21 years, the multivariate RR of gout for men who had gained 30 lb or more since age 21 years was 1.99 (95% CI, 1.49-2.66). In contrast, the multivariate RR for men who had lost 10 lb or more since the study baseline was 0.61 (95% CI, 0.40-0.92). The multivariate RRs of gout were 2.31 (95% CI, 1.96-2.72) for the presence of hypertension and 1.77 (95% CI, 1.42-2.20) for diuretic use.

CONCLUSIONS:

Higher adiposity and weight gain are strong risk factors for gout in men, while weight loss is protective. Hypertension and diuretic use are also important independent risk factors for gout.

Goutbusters Tip #8

Following on from point #7, you should create your own exercise programme. Even if it's something low impact such as 30 minutes of walking a day, you should get in motion and burn off any excess pounds (NB – if you're not sure where to start, or you have other existing health conditions, then please consult with your doctor first).

TIP: as an extra motivational tool, buy a set of new clothes in the new size you want to become. Maybe a size smaller than what you are at the moment.

This is very important – make sure you hang these new clothes in a prominent place in your house, for example on your bedroom door, so that you can see them all the time. Why do I suggest this? Simple, because it's a constant reminder of what you want to become, the idea being that your gout attacks should decrease as your weight decreases...

Now for perhaps the most important tip of all, which is on page 215...

THE BOTTOM LINE: A diet high in meat and seafoods increases the risk of gout, whilst a diet high in dairy products is protective. A moderate intake of purine-rich vegetables or protein is not associated with an increased risk of gout.

Susan J Lee, Robert A Terkeltaub, Arthur Kavanaugh. (2006) Recent developments in diet and gout. Current Opinion in Rheumatology 18:2, 193-198

Choi HK, Atkinson K, Karlson EW, Willett W, Curhan G. Purine-rich foods, dairy and protein intake, and the risk of gout in men. N Engl J Med. 2004;350:1093–103.

Abstract

BACKGROUND:
Various purine-rich foods and high protein intake have long been thought to be risk factors for gout. Similarly, the possibility that the consumption of dairy products has a role in protecting against gout has been raised by metabolic studies. We prospectively investigated the association of these dietary factors with new cases of gout.

METHODS:
Over a 12-year period, we prospectively examined the relationship between purported dietary risk factors and new cases of gout among 47,150 men who had no history of gout at baseline. We used a supplementary questionnaire to ascertain whether participants met the American College of Rheumatology survey criteria for gout. Diet was assessed every four years by means of a food-frequency questionnaire.

RESULTS:
During the 12 years of the study, we documented 730 confirmed new cases of gout.

The multivariate relative risk of gout among men in the highest quintile of meat intake, as compared with those in the lowest quintile, was 1.41 (95 percent confidence interval, 1.07 to 1.86; P for trend = 0.02), and the corresponding relative risk associated with seafood intake was 1.51 (95 percent confidence interval, 1.17 to 1.95; P for trend = 0.02).

In contrast, the incidence of gout decreased with increasing intake of dairy products; the multivariate relative risk among men in the highest quintile, as compared with those in the lowest quintile, was 0.56 (95 percent confidence interval, 0.42 to 0.74; P for trend <0.001). The level of consumption of purine-rich vegetables and the total protein intake were not associated with an increased risk of gout.

CONCLUSIONS:
Higher levels of meat and seafood consumption are associated with an increased risk of gout, whereas a higher level of consumption of dairy products is associated with a decreased risk. Moderate intake of purine-rich vegetables or protein is not associated with an increased risk of gout.

THE BOTTOM LINE: Gout is much more common in, but not exclusive to, men. More research is needed to find out why this is so.

De Souza AW, Fernandes V, Ferrari AJ. Female gout: clinical and laboratory features. J Rheumatol. 2005;32:2186–8.

Abstract

Clinically, gout is generally considered as a preferential male disease. However, it definitely does not occur exclusively in males.

Our aim was to assess differences in the clinical features of gout arthritis between female and male patients. Five electronic databases were searched to identify relevant original studies published between 1977 and 2007.

The included studies had to focus on adult patients with primary gout arthritis and on sex differences in clinical features. Two reviewers independently assessed eligibility and quality of the studies.

Out of 355 articles, 14 were selected. Nine fulfilled the quality and score criteria. We identified the following sex differences in the clinical features of gout in women compared to men: the onset of gout occurs at a higher age, more comorbidity with hypertension or renal insufficiency, more often use of diuretics, less likely to drink alcohol, less often podagra but more often involvement of other joints, less frequent recurrent attacks.

We found interesting sex differences regarding the clinical features of patients with gout arthritis. To diagnose gout in women, knowledge of these differences is essential, and more research is needed to understand and explain the differences, especially in the general population.

THE BOTTOM LINE: Why it's important to keep blood levels of uric acid low in patients with chronic gout in order to prevent further attacks.

Wallace SL, Robinson H, Masi AT, Decker JL, McCarty DJ, Yu TF. Preliminary criteria for the classification of the acute arthritis of primary gout. Arthritis Rheum. 1977;20:895–900.

Rigby AS, Wood PH. Serum uric acid levels and gout: what does this herald for the population?. Clin Exp Rheumatol. 1994;12:395–400.

McCarty DJ. Gout without hyperuricemia. JAMA. 1994;271:302–3.

Terkeltaub RA. Clinical practice. Gout. N Engl J Med. 2003;349:1647–55.

Altman RD, Honig S, Levin JM, Lightfoot RW. Ketoprofen versus indomethacin in patients with acute gouty arthritis: a multicenter, double blind comparative study. J Rheumatol. 1988;15:1422–6.

Shrestha M, Morgan DL, Moreden JM, Singh R, Nelson M, Hayes JE. Randomized double-blind comparison of the analgesic efficacy of intramuscular ketorolac and oral indomethacin in the treatment of acute gouty arthritis. Ann Emerg Med. 1995;26:682–6.

Groff GD, Franck WA, Raddatz DA. Systemic steroid therapy for acute gout: a clinical trial and review of the literature. Semin Arthritis Rheum. 1990;19:329–36.

Schlesinger N, Schumacher R, Catton M, Maxwell L. Colchicine for acute gout. Cochrane Database Syst Rev. 2006;(4):CD006190.

Gutman AB. The past four decades of progress in the knowledge of gout, with an assessment of the present status. Arthritis Rheum. 1973;16:431–45.

Hande KR, Noone RM, Stone WJ. Severe allopurinol toxicity. Description and guidelines for prevention in patients with renal insufficiency. Am J Med. 1984;76:47–56.

Borstad GC, Bryant LR, Abel MP, Scroggie DA, Harris MD, Alloway JA. Colchicine for prophylaxis of acute flares when initiating allopurinol for chronic gouty arthritis. J Rheumatol. 2004;31:2429–32.

Li-Yu J, Clayburne G, Sieck M, Beutler A, Rull M, Eisner E, et al. Treatment of chronic gout. Can we determine when urate stores are depleted enough to prevent attacks of gout?. J Rheumatol. 2001;28:577–80.

Abstract

OBJECTIVE:
To determine if lowering of serum uric acid (SUA) concentrations below 6 mg/dl or longer duration of lowered SUA will result in depletion of urate crystals from the knee joints and prevent further attacks of gout.

METHODS:
A prospective study was initiated 10 years ago at Philadelphia VA Medical Center to attempt to maintain SUA levels of patients with crystal proven gout at < 6.0 mg/dl.

We recalled all 57 patients who were available during 1999. Patients were divided into two groups: Group A, with SUA still > 6 mg/dl, and Group B, with SUA < or = 6 mg/dl.

A knee joint aspirate was requested from all asymptomatic Group B patients and many in Group A. Aspirates were examined by polarised light microscopy for identification of crystals.

RESULTS:
There were no differences between the groups in age, sex, duration of gout, or serum creatinine.

Group A (n = 38) had a mean of six attacks of gout for the recent year, those with tophi having the most frequent attacks. Among the 16 patients in this group who agreed to knee aspiration, monosodium urate (MSU) crystals were found in 14, although they were asymptomatic at the time.

Nineteen patients (Group B) were able to maintain serum urate levels < or = 6 mg/dl for > 12 months. Nearly half of them had no attack of gout for two or more years, with a mean of one attack in the last year for the whole group.

Three patients in whom tophi were found did not have major flares of gout within the past year. Knee joint aspiration was done on 16 asymptomatic patients. Seven (44%) still had MSU crystals present in their knees.

Patients in this group who were taking prophylactic colchicine did not differ with respect to the character of synovial fluid from those who had discontinued it for up to several years, although the frequency of attacks was less in those who continued colchicine.

CONCLUSION:
A majority of patients were able to deplete urate crystal stores in their knee joint fluids when their SUA levels were kept to < or = 6 mg/dl for several years. The mechanisms for persistence in some patients, and whether such crystals have clinical implications, are not known. Patients with chronic gout need serum urate concentrations to be kept low to prevent further attacks.

THE BOTTOM LINE: Massage therapy is effective in gout.

Fam AG, Dunne SM, Iazzetta J, Paton TW. Efficacy and safety of desensitization to allopurinol following cutaneous reactions. Arthritis Rheum. 2001;44:231–8.

Schumacher HR Jr, Chen LX. Newer therapeutic approaches: gout. Rheum Dis Clin North Am. 2006;32:235–44.

Becker MA, Schumacher HR Jr, Wortmann RL, MacDonald PA, Eustace D, Palo WA, et al. Febuxostat compared with allopurinol in patients with hyperuricemia and gout. N Engl J Med. 2005;353:2450–61.

Vogt B. Urate oxidase (rasburicase) for treatment of severe tophaceous gout. Nephrol Dial Transplant. 2005;20:431–3.

Ganson NJ, Kelly SJ, Scarlett E, Sundy JS, Hershfield MS. Control of hyperuricemia in subjects with refractory gout, and induction of antibody against poly(ethylene glycol) (PEG), in a phase I trial of subcutaneous PEGylated urate oxidase. Arthritis Res Ther. 2006;8:R12.

Adam I. Perlman, MD, MPH; Alyse Sabina, MD; Anna-Leila Williams, PA-C, MPH; Valentine Yanchou Njike, MD; David L. Katz, MD, MPH. Massage Therapy for Osteoarthritis of the Knee. A Randomized Controlled Trial. Arch Intern Med. 2006;166:2533-2538

BACKGROUND:
Massage therapy is an attractive treatment option for osteoarthritis (OA), but its efficacy is uncertain. We conducted a randomised, controlled trial of massage therapy for OA of the knee.

METHODS:
Sixty-eight adults with radiographically confirmed OA of the knee were assigned either to treatment (twice-weekly sessions of standard Swedish massage in weeks one to four and once-weekly sessions in weeks five to eight) or to control (delayed intervention). Primary outcomes were changes in the Western Ontario and McMaster Universities Osteoarthritis Index (WOMAC) pain and functional scores

and the visual analog scale of pain assessment. The sample provided 80% statistical power to detect a 20-point difference between groups in the change from baseline on the WOMAC and visual analog scale, with a 2-tailed of .05.

RESULTS:

The group receiving massage therapy demonstrated significant improvements in the mean (SD) WOMAC global scores (−17.44 [23.61] mm; P .001), pain (−18.36 [23.28]; P .001), stiffness (−16.63 [28.82] mm; P .001), and physical function domains (−17.27 [24.36] mm; P .001) and in the visual analog scale of pain assessment (−19.38 [28.16] mm; P .001), range of motion in degrees (3.57 [13.61]; P=.03), and time to walk 50 ft (15 m) in seconds (−1.77 [2.73]; P .01). Findings were unchanged in multivariable models controlling for demographic factors.

CONCLUSIONS:

Massage therapy seems to be efficacious in the treatment of OA of the knee. Further study of cost effectiveness and duration of treatment effect is clearly warranted.

A scientific paper on the importance of urate-lowering treatments related to gout pain relief.

Perez-Ruiz, F. Treating to target: a strategy to cure gout. Rheumatology (2009) 48 (suppl 2): ii9-ii14. doi: 10.1093/rheumatology/kep087

Abstract

Acute gout attacks and the long-term complications of gout are associated with the deposition of monosodium urate (MSU) monohydrate crystals in the joints and soft tissues, causing acute and chronic inflammation.

The aim of long-term treatment is to reduce the serum urate (sUA) level to 6 mg/dl (<360 µmol/l), below the saturation point of MSU, so that new crystals cannot form and existing crystals are dissolved. Serial joint aspiration studies confirmed the disappearance of crystals with effective urate-lowering therapy.

There is good evidence that achieving sUA <6 mg/dl (360 µmol/l) results in freedom from acute gout attacks, and shrinkage and eventual disappearance of tophi.

Gout patients must be informed about their diagnosis and educated about gout management including the importance of compliance with long-term treatment.

Patients starting urate-lowering therapy need to understand the importance of prophylactic therapy with colchicine or NSAIDs to reduce the risk of 'mobilisation flares' in the first few months. In the long term, reduction in the sUA below the target level will result in gout being effectively cured.

Introduction

As already discussed in the first paper in this supplement [1], gout is one of the most common inflammatory arthritic diseases.

It is a true crystal deposition disease and both acute episodes of inflammation (the so-called gout flares or attacks) and the long-term sequelae due to chronic inflammation of gout are induced by monosodium urate (MSU) monohydrate crystals formed in the tissues.

If there are no MSU crystals present, gout cannot occur. This means that if the tissue environment urate concentration is reduced sufficiently, existing crystals are dissolved and new crystals can no longer form, which essentially cures gout.

This potential for cure with adequate long-term treatment makes gout a rewarding condition for clinicians to manage.

This paper will discuss the role of MSU crystals in the pathogenesis of acute and chronic gout and the importance of targeting a low serum urate (sUA) level during the treatment of chronic gout, in order to achieve the clinical benefits of freedom from acute gout attacks, resolution of tophi and prevention of structural damage to joints and tissues.

Practical aspects of the long-term management of gout patients are also reviewed.

Hyperuricaemia as the underlying cause

It is clear that long-standing hyperuricaemia is the principal factor in the occurrence of gout, based not only on the epidemiological evidence, but also on physicochemical principles.

Uric acid is a weak acid that is present in plasma as MSU. Numerous studies have shown that the solubility of MSU is strongly temperature dependent and that the saturation threshold at 37°C is ~ 6.8 mg/dl (408 μmol/l) [2].

However, only a small proportion of patients with hyperuricaemia develop gout and hence other factors must determine whether crystal formation occurs. Several groups have shown that SF from gout patients enhances the formation of MSU crystals [3, 4].

In one study, the addition of SF from gout patients to super-saturated solutions of sodium urate under physiological conditions greatly enhanced crystal formation, whereas SF from OA patients had a modest effect and fluid from RA patients had little effect [3].

Crystals are present, and may be retrieved by aspirating the SF of gout patients during gout flares, but also during asymptomatic (intercritical) periods [5].

However, no correlation has been observed between the size, shape and numbers of crystals in the SF and the severity of inflammation— some patients with severe acute gout may have only a few crystals. Hence, other factors must affect the severity of the inflammatory response in gout [6].

Formation of crystals may initially start in the joint cartilage in an orderly way, suggesting epitaxial nucleation and growth [7].

Acute gout flares

Deposition of crystals may continue for months or years without causing symptoms [8], until shedding of crystals into the SF triggers the first episode of acute gout. Innate immunity (through toll-like receptors) may be involved in MSU-induced macrophage activation [9].

MSU crystals are intensely inflammatory and recent research has provided new insights into the inflammatory process. MSU crystals are phagocytosed by monocytes and macrophages, activating the NALP3 inflammasome and triggering the release of IL-1 and other cytokines. This leads to infiltration of neutrophils and the symptoms of an acute flare [10–12].

Acute gout attacks typically resolve spontaneously and differentiated macrophages, through secretion of TGF-β, may exert a protective role to the joint [13].

Chronic gout

Long-standing persistence of MSU crystals may also cause chronic neutrophilic inflammation [14], osteoclast activation [15] and chronic granulomatous infiltration of the synovium. Micro-aggregates of MSU crystals occur in all patients with gout, but in some, macroscopic aggregates occur, manifested as tophus formation.

Tophi are usually considered to be a late manifestation of gout.

However, intra-articular tophi have been reported before an acute gout attack has occurred [16]. Recent imaging studies have highlighted the presence of asymptomatic tophi not apparent on physical examination [17].

In a recent ultrasound study of patients with asymptomatic hyperuricaemia, tophi were detected in the tendons, synovial membrane or soft tissues in 12 of the 35 examined (34%). Power Doppler showed evidence of inflammation in two-thirds of these [8].

As well as diagnosing tophi, ultrasound can also be useful to detect the deposition of urate crystals on the articular cartilage [18]. MRI and CT are also valuable for detecting asymptomatic tophi [17].

Target sUA in chronic gout

Since it is clear that gout is the consequence of the accumulation of uric acid in the body, the logical way to treat the condition is to lower the sUA level and deplete the body urate pool.

The clinical manifestations of gout are due to deposition of MSU crystals and if the crystals are dissolved completely and no new crystals can form, then the condition is cured. To achieve this, the sUA (and hence the tissue and joint uric acid levels) must be reduced below the saturation point of MSU under physiological conditions.

This has been recognised in recent evidence-based recommendations from the European League against Rheumatism (EULAR) Task Force for Gout, which recommend that the sUA should be reduced to a target of <6 mg/dl (360 µmol/l) [19].

The authors of the recommendations point out that the target sUA level should be linked to the saturation level of MSU rather than to the normal laboratory range, which can vary between populations and with time.

It is also acknowledged in the guidelines that the target sUA may vary depending on the characteristics of the patient and a lower target may be appropriate in patients with extensive crystal deposition.

Goutbusters* Tip #9: Special Free Gift From The Authors Of *Goutbusters

To help you get even more value from this book, please take advantage of the FREE extra resource waiting for you at:

www.drgout.com

Automatic membership to
The Dr Gout Digest FREE enewsletter service

The Dr Gout Digest is your weekly email newsletter service, written exclusively for gout sufferers and those who love them.

Sent to you every Friday, each issue of ***The Dr Gout Digest*** contains details of the latest tips, techniques and strategies to help you relieve your gout pain, and shows you the medical breakthroughs the top health professionals worldwide use to make your life that little bit easier – and more gout free.

When it comes to getting rid of gout pain, you'll get to see what works best, what to avoid, and how to enjoy maximum pain relief in minimum time. And (most important of all) how you can conquer your gout attacks, regain control of your life, health and happiness, and enjoy yourself in the process...

**Here's How To Activate Your Free Membership Of
The Dr Gout Digest enewsletter**

1. Please go to the website at: www.drgout.com

2. Simply complete your name, address and email details in the spaces provided on this webpage.

Continued on the next page...

3. Once we receive these, you'll receive a confirmation email in your inbox. Just following the simple instructions in this email and your membership of *The Dr Gout Digest* enewsletter will be activated automatically.

4. **EXTRA MYSTERY BONUS GIFT**: when you activate your membership, you'll also receive an extra bonus gift (worth £10.00) and only available to members of *The Dr Gout Digest* enewsletter. Full details of how to obtain this when you join...

Go to page 234 for the final tip...

The British Society of Rheumatology (BSR) has also published guidelines for the management of gout and these recommend a stricter sUA target of <5 mg/dl (<300 µmol/l) [20].

Outcome measures

The aim of treatment is to dissolve the crystals, leading to freedom from acute attacks of gout, reduction and disappearance of tophi and prevention of further tissue damage [21].

In the study by Pascual and Sivera [22], arthrocentesis was performed in 18 patients before the initiation of urate-lowering therapy with benzbromarone or allopurinol plus benzbromarone, which are highly effective treatments.

The process was repeated every three months and it was found that crystals soon disappeared from the SF after the dramatic reduction in sUA [22]. The median sUA fell from 9.2 mg/dl (550 µmol/l) before the start of treatment to 4.8 mg/dl (290 µmol/l) after three months of treatment. The time required for the disappearance of urate crystals ranged from 3 to 33 months and was correlated with the duration of gout (rs = 0.71, P < 0.01).

Studies have consistently shown a relationship between sUA levels and the risk of gout flares, providing compelling evidence for targeting low sUA levels.

In a retrospective study of 267 patients, 87% of whom received urate-lowering therapy, there was a strong correlation between the average sUA level and the recurrence of gout attacks: logistic regression analysis showed that the lower the sUA, the less likely the patient was to experience an acute attack (P < 0.001).

The mean sUA in treated patients who experienced gout attacks (n = 69) was 7.01 mg/dl (420 µmol/l) compared with 6.36 mg/dl (388 µmol/l) in those who were free of attacks (n = 163) [23]. In another study, patients with sUA >6 mg/dl (>360 µmol/l) experienced a mean of six attacks of gout in the previous year and MSU crystals were present in 14 of 16 patients on joint aspiration.

In contrast, the group with sUA levels <6 mg/dl (<360 µmol/l) for at least 12 months experienced a mean of one attack in the previous year and almost half had not experienced an attack for two years [24].

These findings were confirmed in a prospective study in 36 patients, which showed that **gout** flares were almost completely eliminated by the second year of urate-lowering therapy targeting the reduction of sUA <6 mg/dl (360 µmol/l). The mean number of flares was 3.4 (± 1.62) per patient-year in the year before the initiation of therapy, 0.93 (± 1.16) in the first year and 0.06 (± 0.25) in the second year of treatment [25].

Maintaining the sUA level at <6 mg/dl (360 µmol/l) also results in a reduction in tophus size. In 14 patients with a gout diagnosis confirmed by the presence of crystals, who underwent ultrasound examination before and after 12 months of urate-lowering therapy, there was an inverse correlation between the mean reduction in the maximal tophus diameter and the average sUA level.

There was a similar inverse correlation between change in tophus volume and sUA levels [26]. These results are in contrast with old studies suggesting that sUA levels did not have an impact on the progression of gout [27], but a careful review of the results shows that sUA levels in these series were not targeted to <6 mg/dl (360 µmol/l), and most patients did not show 'subsaturating' urate levels [27]. Furthermore, the only patient who experienced disappearance of tophi showed sUA levels <4 mg/dl [27].

Some evidence also suggests that the lower the sUA level, the faster the decrease in tophus size, implying that a lower sUA target might be appropriate in patients with severe tophaceous gout [26, 28].

In another study in 63 patients with crystal-proven gout, there was a linear correlation between the sUA level and the speed of reduction of tophus size [28]. This supports the previously suggested concept that existing crystal deposits will be dissolved more quickly at lower sUA levels [29].

In these studies [26, 28], the combination of allopurinol and sulphinpyrazone or allopurinol and benzbromarone resulted in a striking reduction of subcutaneous tophi.

Although not uncommon in the clinical practice of those with a special interest in gout [22, 28], there is no controlled study or long-term follow-up on how to manage combination therapy.

Due to the present restrictions in benzbromarone prescription in the European Union due to liver toxicity concerns, the practical approach would be to consider combination therapy in patients in whom other urate-lowering drugs have not achieved the sUA target for the treatment of gout.

Practical issues in the management of gout patients

It is important that the patients are informed about their diagnosis and educated about gout. It is particularly important to help them understand that MSU crystal observation equals the certainty of the diagnosis and that there is a need for adequate, long-term therapy designed to eradicate the crystals.

It is also essential to explain to the patient about the role of lifestyle changes and non-pharmacological approaches to the management of gout.

Obese patients should lose weight gradually and the diet should be adjusted to avoid an excess intake of proteins from meat and fish (but not proteins of dairy origin) and other high-purine foods.

The intake of alcohol, especially beer, should be reduced to a minimum [19, 20]. While these measures may have a relatively modest effect on the sUA level, they are quite beneficial for the general health of the patient.

Hyperuricaemia is often associated with dyslipidaemia, hypertension, insulin resistance and obesity as part of the metabolic syndrome [30] and hence management of these risk factors should be considered as part of the overall therapeutic approach to gout.

There is no consensus on when to start therapy with urate-lowering drugs. All experts would agree that patients with severe gout (recurrent flares, polyarticular joint involvement, presence of tophi or structural joint involvement) should be encouraged to start a urate-lowering drug.

The issue is whether waiting for severe gout to develop should be considered as good clinical practice. Reference to some studies may help patients and doctors in their decision-making process.

Over 50% of the patients not treated with urate-lowering drugs developed tophaceous X-ray involvement, suggesting that untreated gout is not a mild, non-progressive disease [31].

Severity of gout is also associated with a higher rate of ischaemic heart disease [32], and gout itself, independent from hyperuricaemia and other well-known vascular risk factors, may be associated with an increased risk of myocardial infarction [33].

Furthermore, in a hypothetical decision model analysis, urate-lowering therapy would be cost saving for patients with two or more flares a year, and for patients with one flare a year and at risk of developing adverse events to NSAIDs [34].

With this in mind, patients and doctors should consider carefully the advantages (high rate of success in preventing both flares and the development of severe gout) and the risks (low rate of adverse events due to urate-lowering drugs) when making their decisions.

Once a decision has been taken to start urate-lowering therapy, especially if urate-lowering drugs are needed, it is important that the patient understands that there is a risk of 'mobilisation flares' in the first few months of treatment.

Such flares are thought to be caused by the rapid reduction in sUA after the start of urate-lowering agents or after a change in dose. Acute attacks occur after the initiation of all urate-lowering treatments and it is noteworthy that a high incidence has been observed with pegloticase, which causes a very rapid and dramatic fall in sUA [35].

The EULAR recommendations include initiating urate-lowering drugs at low dose, with step-up increase of dose, if tolerated, to properly control sUA levels [19]. Rapid reduction of sUA to subsaturating levels has been associated with an increase in the risk of gout flares [36–38], so reduction of sUA levels should be as slow as possible [36].

Initiating prophylactic therapy with either low-dose colchicine or an NSAID during the first months of urate-lowering therapy to reduce the risk of acute flares has also been recommended [19].

There have been two randomised controlled trials, published three decades apart, that evaluate the use of colchicine in this way [39, 40].

In one study, in patients being treated with probenecid, the addition of colchicine 1.5 mg/day (0.5 mg three times daily) resulted in a significant reduction in the number of acute attacks in the six-month period (P < 0.05) [39].

In the second trial, prophylaxis with colchicine at a dose of 0.6 mg twice daily for six months during the initiation of allopurinol, significantly reduced the frequency and severity of acute flares (P = 0.008) [40].

The evidence to support the use of NSAIDs is less robust (no trial data available) but these agents are used as an alternative. In all cases, the balance of risks and benefits must be considered [19, 20].

It should be explained to patients that mobilisation flares, if they occur, can be regarded as the 'price to pay' for the cure of gout and that in any case the risk can be reduced with prophylactic therapy.

The patient also needs to understand about the importance of adhering to the prescribed therapy in order to achieve the sUA target and maintain subsaturation sUR levels in the long term to finally eradicate MSU crystals. It is important to monitor sUA levels regularly to ensure that the target is met and also to check on compliance.

As discussed above, long-term urate-lowering therapy to achieve sUA levels <6 mg/dl (360 µmol/l) results in almost complete prevention of acute gout flares.

It is normally recommended that urate-lowering therapy should be continued indefinitely.

However, it is reasonable to ask whether it is possible to withdraw urate-lowering therapy after a long period of sustained control of the sUA, resulting in depletion of the body pool of uric acid.

To answer this question, a prospective observational study was undertaken in patients who had received >5 years of urate-lowering therapy [41]. Patients were followed up for a maximum of six years after withdrawal of urate-lowering therapy and sUA levels were measured regularly during this time.

Patients were stratified according to the median sUA during urate-lowering therapy; the group with mean sUA levels of <5.05 mg/dl (<303 µmol/l) during therapy had a mean period of 49 months without recurrence of gout compared with 34 months in those with higher sUA levels.

Similarly, those with mean sUA levels <8.75 mg/dl (<525 µmol/l) after withdrawal of urate-lowering therapy had a mean period of 47 months without recurrence compared with 34 months in those with higher sUA levels after urate-lowering therapy withdrawal.

This suggests that, following a prolonged period of good control of sUA levels, it may be feasible to withdraw treatment for a period, or at least the sUA control target may be less rigid during the long-term ('crystal formation prevention') period of treatment than during the initial ('crystal depleting') period of treatment.

Management of patients with comorbidities

It is important to consider comorbidities in gout patients [42]. Renal function impairment function should be assessed by estimating creatinine clearance [43] rather than relying on the serum creatinine level.

In patients with renal impairment, the dose of allopurinol must be adjusted according to renal function [44], and some uricosuric drugs may not be effective — such as probenecid and sulphinpyrazone — in patients with moderate renal function impairment, although benzbromarone may still show efficacy, but only at higher doses, in patients with moderate renal function impairment [25].

Severe allopurinol toxicity has been associated with renal function impairment due to the accumulation of oxypurinol, its active metabolite, which is renally excreted [45], and not to a direct toxic effect on the kidneys.

Although genetic predisposition has been recently reported in 100% of the Han Chinese showing Severe Cutaneous Adverse Reactions (SCAR) to allopurinol [46] and in 55% of the patients of European ancestry [47], renal function impairment was the other, highly statistically significant, factor associated with SCAR in patients on allopurinol [46].

In addition, the side effects of colchicine and NSAIDs may be more frequent in patients with renal dysfunction and prescription use should be restricted in renally impaired persons to treat acute flares and for long-term prophylaxis [48].

Conclusions

In summary, gout is a crystal deposition disease that is associated with acute and chronic inflammation.

However, it can be cured by long-term reduction in the sUA level <6 mg/dl (360 µmol/l), sufficient to dissolve crystal deposits and prevent formation of new crystals.

This results in freedom from acute gout attacks, shrinkage and eventual disappearance of tophi and prevention of further tissue damage.

While gout itself can be cured by lowering the sUA level below this target, joint and tissue damage that has already occurred may not be reversible, emphasising the importance of treating the condition before such permanent damage has occurred.

In the author's personal opinion, for all patients except those with very mild gout, the lower the sUA level, the better during the first few years of treatment. However, a level close to the saturation level may be acceptable later on, once the body urate pool has returned to normal and crystal deposition cleared.

Finally, it is important to educate the patient about their disease and the importance of their contribution to (compliance with) long-term treatment.

- *Doherty M. New insights into the epidemiology of gout. Rheumatology 2009;48 Suppl. 2:ii2-8.*

- *Fiddis RW, Vlachos N, Calvert PD. Studies of urate crystallisation in relation to gout. Ann Rheum Dis 1983;42 Suppl. 1:12-15.*

- *Tak HK, Cooper SM, Wilcox WR. Studies on the nucleation of monosodium urate at 37 degrees C. Arthritis Rheum 1980;23:574-80.*

- *McGill NW, Dieppe PA. Evidence for a promoter of urate crystal formation in gouty synovial fluid. Ann Rheum Dis 1991;50:558-61.*

- *Pascual E, Batlle-Gualda E, Martinez A, Rosas J, Vela P. Synovial fluid analysis for diagnosis of intercritical gout. Ann Intern Med 1999;131:756-9.*

- *Antommattei O, Schumacher HR, Reginato AJ, Clayburne G. Prospective study of morphology and phagocytosis of synovial fluid monosodium urate crystals in gouty arthritis. J Rheumatol 1984;11:741-4.*

- *Pascual E, Ordonez S. Orderly arrayed deposit of urate crystals in gout suggest epitaxial formation. Ann Rheum Dis 1998;57:255.*

- *Puig JG, de Miguel E, Castillo MC, Rocha AL, Martinez MA, Torres RJ. Asymptomatic hyperuricemia: impact of ultrasonography. Nucleosides Nucleotides Nucleic Acids 2008;27:592-5.*

- *Liu-Bryan R, Scott P, Sydlaske A, Rose DM, Terkeltaub R. Innate immunity conferred by Toll-like receptors 2 and 4 and myeloid differentiation factor 88 expression is pivotal to monosodium urate monohydrate crystal-induced inflammation. Arthritis Rheum 2005;52:2936-46.*

- *So A. [Recent advances in the pathophysiology of hyperuricemia and gout]. Rev Med Suisse 2007;3:720. 722–4.*

- *Martinon F, Petrilli V, Mayor A, Tardivel A, Tschopp J. Gout-associated uric acid crystals activate the NALP3 inflammasome. Nature 2006;440:237-41.*

- *Petrilli V, Martinon F. The inflammasome, auto-inflammatory diseases, and gout. Joint Bone Spine 2007;74:571-6.*

- *Yagnik DR, Evans BJ, Florey O, Mason JC, Landis RC, Haskard DO. Macrophage release of transforming growth factor beta1 during resolution of monosodium urate monohydrate crystal-induced inflammation. Arthritis Rheum 2004;50:2273-80.*

- *Pascual E. Persistence of monosodium urate crystals and low-grade inflammation in the synovial fluid of patients with untreated gout. Arthritis Rheum 1991;34:141-5.*

- *Dalbeth N, Smith T, Nicolson B, et al. Enhanced osteoclastogenesis in patients with tophaceous gout: urate crystals promote osteoclast development through interactions with stromal cells. Arthritis Rheum 2008;58:1854-65.*

- *Yu KH. Intraarticular tophi in a joint without a previous gouty attack. J Rheumatol 2003;30:1868-70.*

- *Perez-Ruiz F, Naredo E. Imaging modalities and monitoring measures of gout. Curr Opin Rheumatol 2007;19:128-33.*

- *Thiele RG, Schlesinger N. Diagnosis of gout by ultrasound. Rheumatology 2007;46:1116-21.*

- *Zhang W, Doherty M, Bardin T, et al. EULAR evidence based recommendations for gout. Part II: Management. Report of a task force of the EULAR Standing Committee for International Clinical Studies Including Therapeutics (ESCISIT). Ann Rheum Dis 2006;65:1312-24.*

- *Jordan KM, Cameron JS, Snaith M, et al. British Society for Rheumatology and British Health Professionals in Rheumatology guideline for the management of gout. Rheumatology 2007;46:1372-4.*

- *Perez-Ruiz F, Liote F. Lowering serum uric acid levels: what is the optimal target for improving clinical outcomes in gout? Arthritis Rheum 2007;57:1324-8.*

- *CrossRefM, Pascual E, Sivera F. Time required for disappearance of urate crystals from synovial fluid after successful hypouricaemic treatment relates to the duration of gout. Ann Rheum Dis 2007;66:1056-8.*

- *Shoji A, Yamanaka H, Kamatani N. A retrospective study of the relationship between serum urate level and recurrent attacks of gouty arthritis: evidence for reduction of recurrent gouty arthritis with antihyperuricemic therapy. Arthritis Rheum 2004;51:321-5.*

- *Li-Yu J, Clayburne G, Sieck M, et al. Treatment of chronic gout. Can we determine when urate stores are depleted enough to prevent attacks of gout? J Rheumatol 2001;28:577-80.*

- *Perez-Ruiz F, Calabozo M, Fernandez-Lopez MJ, et al. Treatment of chronic gout in patients with renal function impairment: an open, randomized actively controlled study. J Clin Rheumatol 1999;5:49-55.*

- *Perez-Ruiz F, Martin I, Canteli B. Ultrasonographic measurement of tophi as an outcome measure for chronic gout. J Rheumatol 2007;34:1888-93.*

- *McCarthy GM, Barthelemy CR, Veum JA, Wortmann RL. Influence of antihyperuricemic therapy on the clinical and radiographic progression of gout. Arthritis Rheum 1991;34:1489-94.*

- *Perez-Ruiz F, Calabozo M, Pijoan JI, Herrero-Beites AM, Ruibal A. Effect of urate-lowering therapy on the velocity of size reduction of tophi in chronic gout. Arthritis Rheum 2002;47:356-60.*

- *Goldfarb E, Smyth CJ. Effects of allopurinol, a xanthine oxidase inhibitor, and sulfinpyrazone upon the urinary and serum urate concentrations in eight patients with tophaceous gout. Arthritis Rheum 1966;9:414-23.*

- *Puig JG, Martinez MA. Hyperuricemia, gout and the metabolic syndrome. Curr Opin Rheumatol 2008;20:187-91.*

- *Yu TF, Gutman AB. Principles of current management of primary gout. Am J Med Sci 1967;254:893-907.*

- *Chen SY, Chen CL, Shen ML. Severity of gouty arthritis is associated with Q-wave myocardial infarction: a large-scale, cross-sectional study. Clin Rheumatol 2007;26:308-13.*

- *Krishnan E, Baker JF, Furst DE, Schumacher HR. Gout and the risk of acute myocardial infarction. Arthritis Rheum 2006;54:2688-96.*

- *Ferraz MB, O'Brien B. A cost effectiveness analysis of urate lowering drugs in nontophaceous recurrent gouty arthritis. J Rheumatol 1995;22:908-14.*

- *Sundy JS, Ganson NJ, Kelly SJ, et al. Pharmacokinetics and pharmacodynamics of intravenous PEGylated recombinant mammalian urate oxidase in patients with refractory gout. Arthritis Rheum 2007;56:1021-8.*

- *Yamanaka H, Togashi R, Hakoda M, et al. Optimal range of serum urate concentrations to minimize risk of gouty attacks during anti-hyperuricemic treatment. Adv Exp Med Biol 1998;431:13-8.*

- *Becker MA, Schumacher HR Jr, Wortmann RL, et al. Febuxostat compared with allopurinol in patients with hyperuricemia and gout. N Engl J Med 2005;353:2450-61.*

- *Sundy JS, Becker MA, Baraf HS, et al. Reduction of plasma urate levels following treatment with multiple doses of pegloticase (polyethylene glycol-conjugated uricase) in patients with treatment-failure gout: results of a phase II randomized study. Arthritis Rheum 2008;58:2882-91.*

- *Paulus HE, Schlosstein LH, Godfrey RG, Klinenberg JR, Bluestone R. Prophylactic colchicine therapy of intercritical gout. A placebo-controlled study of probenecid-treated patients. Arthritis Rheum 1974;17:609-14.*

- *Borstad GC, Bryant LR, Abel MP, Scroggie DA, Harris MD, Alloway JA. Colchicine for prophylaxis of acute flares when initiating allopurinol for chronic gouty arthritis. J Rheumatol 2004;31:2429-32.*

- *Perez-Ruiz F, Atxotegi J, Hernando I, Calabozo M, Nolla JM. Using serum urate levels to determine the period free of gouty symptoms after withdrawal of long-term urate-lowering therapy: a prospective study. Arthritis Rheum 2006;55:786-90.*

- *Zhang W, Doherty M, Pascual E, et al. EULAR evidence based recommendations for gout. Part I: Diagnosis. Report of a task force of the Standing Committee for International Clinical Studies Including Therapeutics (ESCISIT). Ann Rheum Dis 2006;65:1301-11.*

- *Levey AS, Coresh J, Balk E, et al. National Kidney Foundation practice guidelines for chronic kidney disease: evaluation, classification, and stratification. Ann Intern Med 2003;139:137-47.*

- *Perez-Ruiz F, Hernando I, Villar I, Nolla JM. Correction of allopurinol dosing should be based on clearance of creatinine, but not plasma creatinine levels: another insight to allopurinol-related toxicity. J Clin Rheumatol 2005;11:129-33.*

- *Emmerson BT, Gordon RB, Cross M, Thomson DB. Plasma oxipurinol concentrations during allopurinol therapy. Br J Rheumatol 1987;26:445-9.*

- *Hung SI, Chung WH, Liou LB, et al. HLA-B*5801 allele as a genetic marker for severe cutaneous adverse reactions caused by allopurinol. Proc Natl Acad Sci USA 2005;102:4134-9.*

- *Lonjou C, Borot N, Sekula P, et al. A European study of HLA-B in Stevens-Johnson syndrome and toxic epidermal necrolysis related to five high-risk drugs. Pharmacogenet Genomics 2008;18:99-107.*

- *Perez-Ruiz F, Schlesinger N. Management of gout. Scand J Rheumatol 2008;37:81-9.*

British Society for Rheumatology and British Health Professionals in Rheumatology Guideline for the Management of Gout

Jordan KM, Cameron JS, Snaith M, Zhang W, Doherty M, Seckl J, et al. British Society for Rheumatology and British Health Professionals in Rheumatology Standards, Guidelines and Audit Working Group (SGAWG). British Society for Rheumatology and British Health Professionals in Rheumatology guideline for the management of gout. Rheumatol (Oxford)2007;46:1372-4:

Scope and purpose of the guideline

Gout is a common disease both in primary care and hospital practice. Although drug therapy for gout has become a paradigm for the effective management and prevention of an acute and potentially chronic rheumatic disease, many of the recommendations for treatment are based on expert consensus rather than research evidence and audits of practice suggest that treatment is very variable.

Guideline for the management of gout

This is a short summary of the guideline. The full guideline can be accessed at Rheumatology Online (www.rheumatology. oxfordjournals.org).

The management pathways proposed are summarised in the accompanying flowchart. The strength recommendations, based on levels of evidence, are graded A–C, and the recommendations are divided into three sections:

Management of acute gout

1. Affected joints should be rested (C) and analgesic, anti-inflammatory drug therapy commenced immediately, and continued for one to two weeks (A).

2. Fast-acting oral NSAIDs at maximum doses are the drugs of choice when there are no contraindications (A).

3. In patients with increased risk of peptic ulcers, bleeds or perforations, co-prescription of gastro-protective agents should follow standard guidelines for the use of NSAIDs and Coxibs (A).

4. Colchicine can be an effective alternative but is slower to work than NSAIDs (A). In order to diminish the risks of adverse effects (especially diarrhoea) it should be used in doses of 500 µg bd–qds (C).

5. Allopurinol should not be commenced during an acute attack (B) but in patients already established on allopurinol, it should be continued and the acute attack should be treated conventionally (A).

6. Opiate analgesics can be used as adjuncts (C).

7. Intra-articular corticosteroids are highly effective in acute gouty monoarthritis (B) and i.a, oral, i.m or i.v corticosteroids can be effective in patients unable to tolerate NSAIDs, and in patients refractory to other treatments (A).

8. If diuretc drugs are being used to treat hypertension, an alternative antihypertensive agent should be considered, but in patients with heart failure, diuretic therapy should not be discontinued (C).

Recommendations for diet, lifestyle modification and non-pharmacological modalities of therapy

1. In overweight patients, dietary modification to achieve ideal body weight should be attempted (B), but 'crash dieting' (B) and high protein/low carbohydrate (Atkins-type) diets (C) should be avoided.

2. Inclusion of skimmed milk and/or low fat yoghurt, soy beans and vegetable sources of protein and cherries, in the diet should be encouraged (B).

3. Intake of high purine foods and red meat should be restricted (B). Liver, kidneys, shellfish and yeast extracts should be avoided (B), and overall protein intake should be restricted (C).

4. Patients with gout and a history of urolithiasis should be encouraged to drink >2 l of water daily (B) and avoid dehydration (C). Alkalinisation of the urine with potassium citrate (60 mEq/day) should be considered in recurrent stone formers (B).

5. Alcohol consumption should be restricted to <21 units/week (men) and 14 units/week (women) (B), and patients should be encouraged to have at least three alcohol-free days per week (C). Beer, stout, port and similar fortified wines are best avoided (C).

6. Patients should be discouraged from undertaking trials of herbal remedies without medical consultation (C).

7. Affected joints should be elevated and exposed in a cool environment (C). 'Bed cages' (C) and ice packs (B) can be effective adjuncts to therapy.

8. Trauma to joints (B) and intense physical exercise (B) should be avoided but moderate physical exercise encouraged (B).

Management of recurrent, intercritical and chronic gout

1. The plasma urate should be maintained below, 300 μmol/l (C).

2. In uncomplicated gout uric acid lowering drug therapy should be started if a second attack, or further attacks occur within one yr (B).

3. Uric acid lowering drug therapy should also be offered to patients with tophi (C), patients with renal insufficiency (B) patients with uric acid stones and gout (B) and to patients who need to continue treatment with diuretics (B).

4. Commencement of uric acid-lowering drug therapy should be delayed until one to two weeks after inflammation has settled (C).

5. Initial long-term treatment of recurrent uncomplicated gout normally should be with allopurinol starting in a dose of 50–100 mg/day and increasing by 50–100 mg increments every

few weeks, adjusted if necessary for renal function, until the therapeutic target (SUA <300 µmol/l) is reached (maximum dose 900 mg) (B).

6. Uricosuric agents can be used as second-line drugs in patients who are under-excretors of uric acid and in those resistant to, or intolerant of, allopurinol (B). The preferred drugs are sulphinpyrazone (200–800 mg/day) in patients with normal renal function or benzbromarone (50–200 mg/day) in patients with mild/moderate renal insufficiency (B).

7. Colchicine 0.5 mg bd should be co-prescribed following initiation of treatment with allopurinol or uricosuric drugs, and continued for up to 6 months (A). In patients who cannot tolerate colchicine, an NSAID or Coxib can be substituted provided that there are no contraindications, but the duration of NSAID or Coxib cover should be limited to 6 weeks (C).

8. Aspirin in low doses (75–150 mg/day) has insignificant effects on the plasma urate, and should be used as required for cardiovascular prophylaxis (B). However, aspirin in analgesic doses (600–2400 mg/day) interferes with uric acid excretion and should be avoided (B).

The full guideline also contains recommendations for the use of uricolytic agents and combined therapy with allopurinol and uricosuric drugs; as well as for the management of special groups of patients with chronic gout.

****

The previous guideline has been developed as a National Guideline, acceptable for use throughout the NHS in the UK.

If followed and implemented, these guidelines will provide an opportunity to improve the quality of care for patients with gout in both hospital and community settings.

> **Goutbusters Tip #10**
>
> If and when you suffer a gout attack, then re-read **Goutbusters**, and the answer to your gout pain will – hopefully – be at your fingertips. If in doubt, or if symptoms persist, please consult your doctor.